"I Feel Your Pain!"

Best,

[signature]

Also by Doug Marlette

"I FEEL YOUR PAIN!"

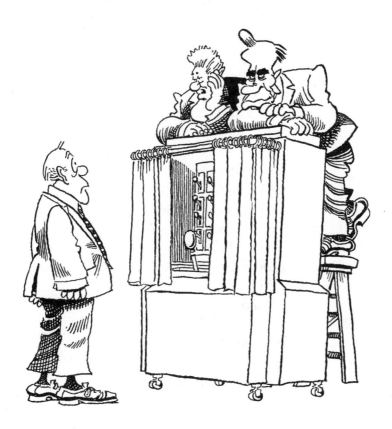

Doug Marlette

🌲 Loblolly Books
Winston-Salem, North Carolina

Published by:
Loblolly Books
716 Archer Rd.
Winston-Salem, NC 27106
(910) 774-6600

**Additional autographed and personalized
copies of this book are available from the
publisher at the above address or by calling:
Toll free (888) LOBLOLLY.**

Manufactured in the United States of America.

ISBN 0-9654505-0-3

Library of Congress Catalog Card Number: 96-78288

Book design by Stephen Berry
Cover design by Patrick Berry and Ron W. Lim
Cover art by Doug Marlette
Cover color by Adam Cohen
Cover photo by Erica Berger

98 97 96   5 4 3 2 1

To my brother, Chris Marlette,
The very finest of teachers, coaches, fathers,
friends, and brothers.

And in memory of Judge James B. MacMillan,
who showed us all the way.

Acknowledgments

With love and gratitude as always to:
Melinda and Jackson Marlette

And many thanks to:
Peggy, Andy, and Kristen Marlette, Elmer and Marie Marlette, Marianne and Terry Neal, and Will Kiker

Pat Conroy, artist, warrior, brother, twin, mirror, friend, exposed nerve ending, whose love of language and art bleeds through his pores

Ted Teague, who made this book possible and to all the folks at Loblolly Books, Steve Berry, whose eye and editorial skills were indispensable, Adam Cohen, esteemed colleague and *Herschel* cartoonist, for his color sense and Mac wisdom, and Patrick Berry, for coming through in the pinch

Will Blythe, an editor of uncommon grace, open heart, and swashbuckling spirit, with the ideal combination of New York mind and Southern gentility

Erica Berger, fellow picture person, New York survivor, and photographer extraordinaire

Marly Rusoff, for her advice and friendship

And to all my friends and colleagues at Newsday, our steadfast publisher, Ray Jansen, editorial page editor Jim Klurfeld, Carol Richards, Noel Rubinton, Joe Dolman, Pat Stewart, Andrea DeJohn, Diane Daniels, and the entire Viewpoints staff, Tony Marro, Howie Schneider, Jim Toedtman, and the Washington Bureau, the Newsday library and everyone who fields all my whacky photo requests, especially Peggy Lundquist, Kathryn Sweeney and Lesley Coven, and all my fellow early risers in the New York office: Bill Reel, who's almost converted me to Catholicism, Linda Winer, my favorite theater critic, Murray Kempton, who keeps on keeping on, and to the memory of our valiant New York Newday staff.

Foreword

by Pat Conroy

Doug Marlette is a prince of mayhem and unrest who has spent his entire adult life drawing pictures that unnerve the populace, eviscerate the arrogant, and create fault lines running through the aisles of serenity itself. He is a political cartoonist of the first rank, has a Pulitzer Prize to prove it, and you would not wish to wake up one morning and stare at a caricature of yourself drawn by Marlette's savage and unsparing eye. He draws so well and so wickedly that he can make even physical beauty look like a crime against nature. If Marlette draws your face for public consumption, it would be hard ever to stare into a mirror again without breaking into tears or laughter. When I met President Clinton, he looked like a man granted conditional leave from a Marlette cartoon to run the country. Doug Marlette does not just draw; he defines, nails it down, then sets it in stone. He is the best daily political cartoonist now working in this country and the competition is fierce. He is the leading light in a very golden age of graphic satire.

But the political cartoonist is one of the oddest ducks in the menagerie of art. There is something overripe, overdone, overarching, and over-reaching about this bizarre and necessary art form. With political cartoonists exaggeration becomes a form of resistance to spin and manipulation, almost an act of modesty. His task is to make grotesquerie visible to both the human eye and the funny bone. Even when the cartoonist provokes great laughter you are aware of the awful coughing of blood in the back room and the mortician's number written on the wallpaper above the phone. He is the luckiest of artists because restraint and good taste rarely have to be yielded to. His is the art of the cruel. But the greatest of these cartoonists, like Marlette, rarely make an error of judgment.

Everything that Daumier or Goya had to consider in the composition of a painting, Doug Marlette and his tribe must consider in their daily assault on the beaches of America's newspapers. There is modulation, restraint, and craft in the artistry, but this is often hidden beneath the knockout punch of the message itself. The political cartoonist does not flatter with his portraiture, but reduces all body parts to their barest essences. I never noticed Reagan's wattles, Clinton's jaw, Bush's chin, or Dole's eyebrows until I saw them highlighted again and again in Marlette's cartoons. One of the bravest things an

American politician does is submit himself to the unerring, unprincipled, savage eyes of American political cartoonists. But there is great value here. The caricature is a sketch of the shadow one's soul makes as it crosses the room.

The first book I ever bought my mother as a birthday present was a copy of Herblock's political cartoons from the Washington Post. My parents were aficianados of Herblock's art and would often turn to the editorial page first to get a glimpse of the biles and fevers of Mr. Block's daily take on the world. I learned from looking at Herblock over the years that nuclear bombs had interesting faces, but always needed a shave.

In contrast to Herblock and Marlette, editorial writers are mere one-celled animals who pride themselves on dispassion and a lack of nerve endings. They are enthralled by their own balance, forethought, and measured responses. Not Marlette. In the twenty years I have known him I have never once caught him with his pants down displaying a single, measured response. His is a gift for instant and abiding fury. Where the editorial writer is a toothless spaniel pointing toward the pasture where the quail have long since taken flight, the political cartoonist is the bird hunter with a smoking AK-47. Political cartoonists who make you yawn are soon unemployed or unnoticed. The great ones live to knock your socks off. They live to hit it out of the park. They draw; you bleed.

The political cartoon is my favorite part of the daily newspaper and the only portion I ever clip. I savor the well-drawn image, the one that tells me what I think long before I am even aware of it. It is the one place in a newspaper where lightning is allowed to strike every single day. If the cartoon is on the mark, it can burn a hole in the consciousness of a city. If it is on target, it can change a Republican into a Democrat, a chauvinist into a feminist, a racist into a civil libertarian, a Gore Vidal into a William F. Buckley. The great cartoon is an editorial with rows of teeth like a hammerhead. No one has ever remembered the content or phraseology of a single editorial. The editorial page is often the place where the English language goes to die. If you could bottle the written editorials of most newspapers there would be no need for Sominex. The editorial writer tries to shape your thinking, but the cartoonist admits you to that secret country where you learn how to feel what it is you're supposed to think. The political cartoonist is to the equanimity of newsrooms what the splitting of the atom was to the architecture of Hiroshima. I have never known a cartoonist who was trusted completely by the editorial page editor and that is precisely the reason why the New York Times has never had one and probably never will.

To be a lover of Doug Marlette's art, you have to have fangs and claws and enjoy the smell of fear that chased game give off during the hunt. His game is not for the squeamish or delicate. This is Marlette's glory and this is homage to the First Amendment.

Let me try to define Doug Marlette, the artist who awaits you here, who lies in wait for you. Where I see a beauty queen, Marlette sees the gargoyle beneath the makeup. Where you and I might welcome spring with a fertility dance, Marlette digs up a corpse and fingers its entrails. Where we say the Lord's prayer, Marlette lowcrawls out to the desert to be tempted for forty days and nights by all the Satanic forces loose in the world. His antennae are always up and quivering and moving among both kings and cockroaches, sensitive to the meretricious, the outrageous, the tragicomic, the sublime. Where we see nobility of purpose, Marlette senses outrage and deceit. Where you and I see statesmanship, Marlette smells the foul gases of corruption. We reach for the roses and *eau de colognes* and Marlette grasps instinctively for the clothespin and formaldehyde.

Political cartoonists are the meanest people on earth who function in our society without requiring hospitalization or imprisonment. Yes, Marlette's powers of hatred are greater than ours, but so are his power to love and praise, to exalt and to hold up to reverent honor, as you will see here in his eulogy drawings. Cartoons are fingerprints by which we discover the deepest, most primitive stirrings of our race. Marlette sees terrible things that he must tell to us, beautiful things he must draw for us as well. All of them are lost between abomination and the valentine.

Fasten your seatbelts. Return your tray tables and seat backs to their original upright position. Make sure you listen to all the flight attendant's instructions. You are about to be illustrated and illuminated.

Doug Marlette is waiting for you.

Pat Conroy
Fripp Island, S.C.
August 1996

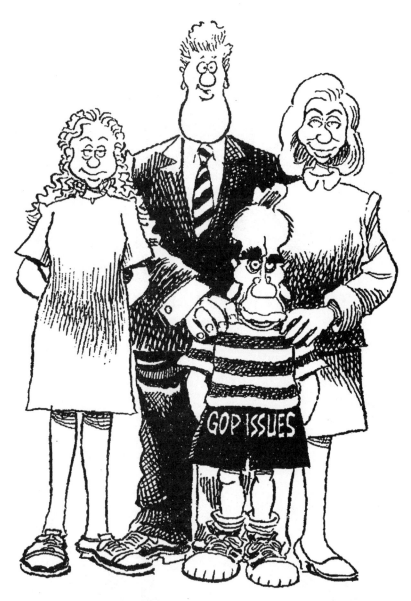

" WE DECIDED TO ADOPT!"

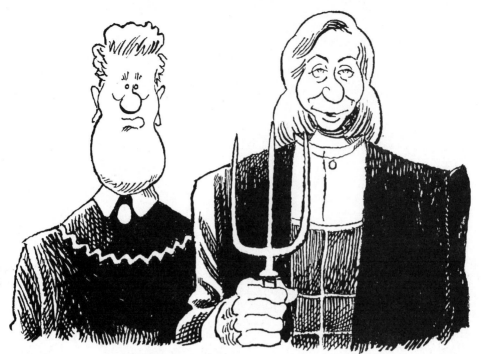

" STAND BY YOUR MAN ! "

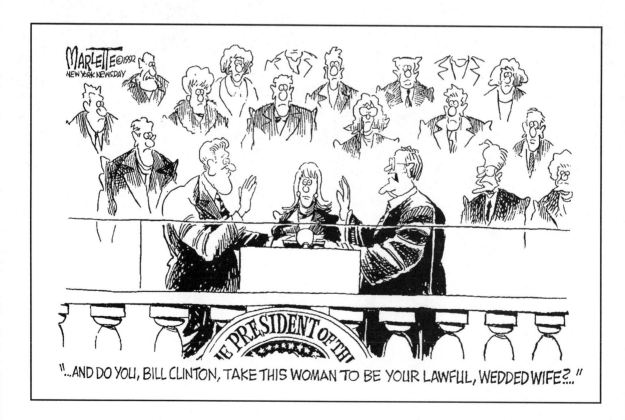

"...AND DO YOU, BILL CLINTON, TAKE THIS WOMAN TO BE YOUR LAWFUL, WEDDED WIFE?..."

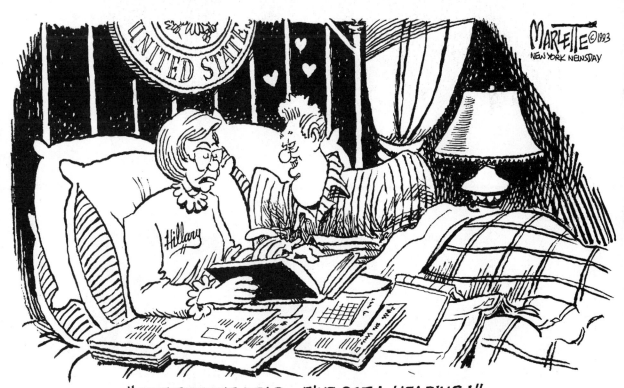

" NOT TONIGHT, DEAR — I'VE GOT A *HEARING!* "

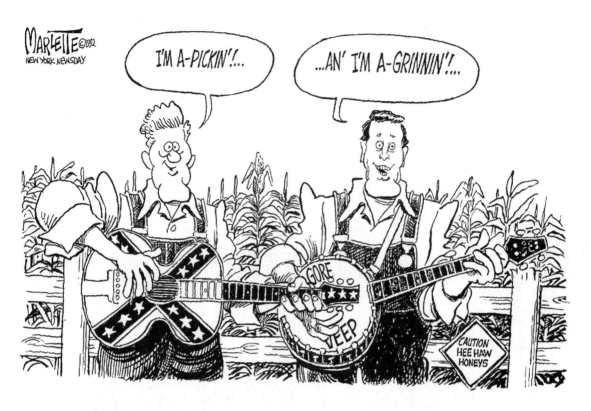

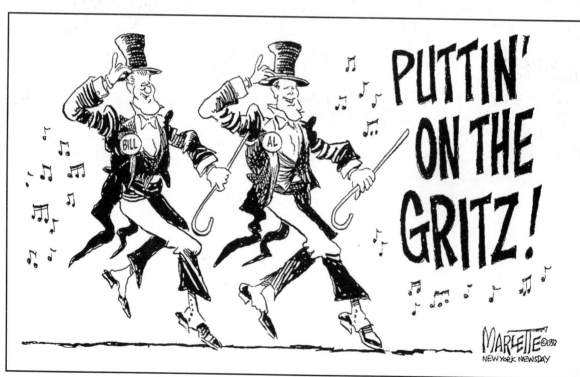

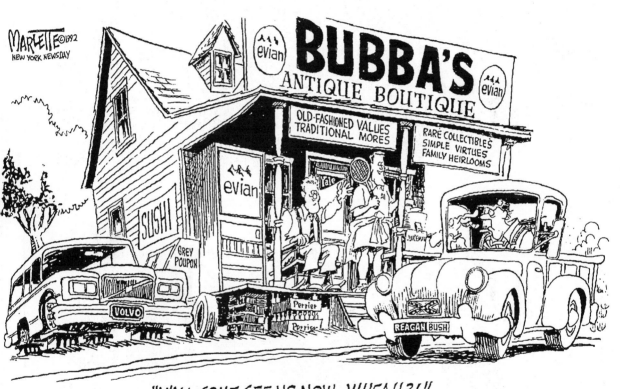

"Y'ALL COME SEE US NOW, Y'HEAH?!"

9

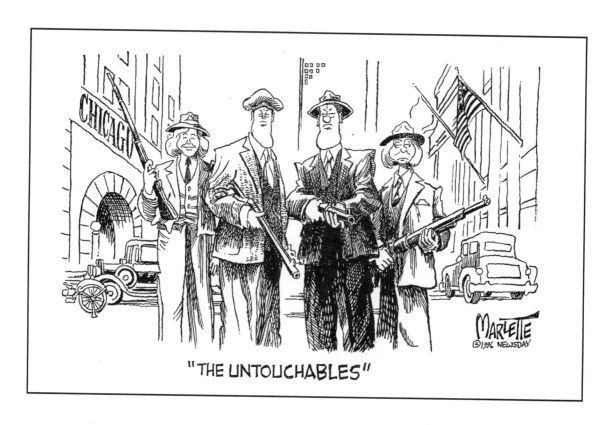

"THE UNTOUCHABLES"

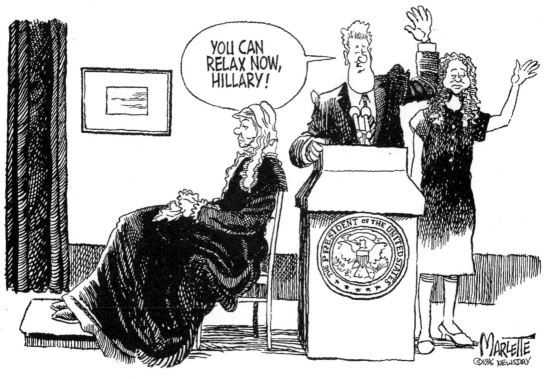

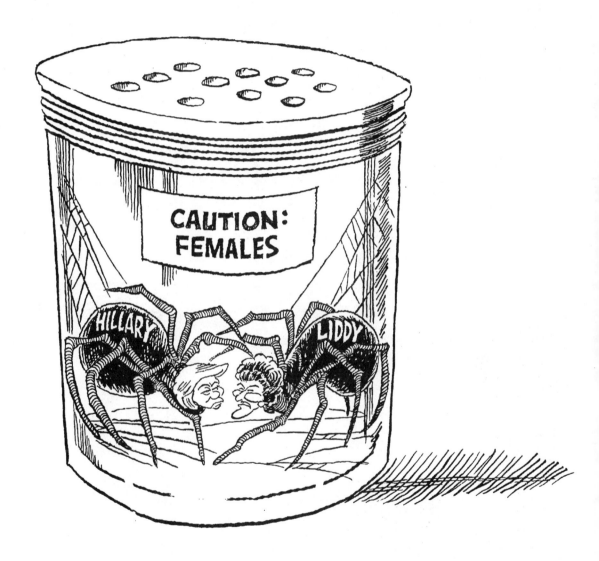

CONVENTION SKETCHBOOK CHICAGO '96...

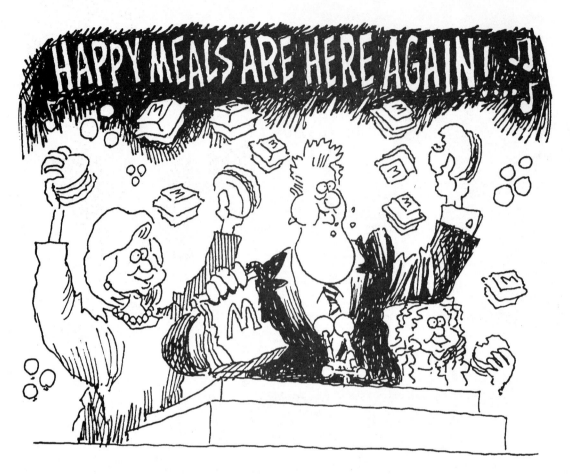

HAPPY MEALS ARE HERE AGAIN! ♪♪

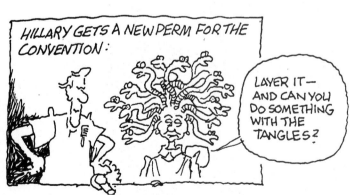

HILLARY GETS A NEW PERM FOR THE CONVENTION:

LAYER IT— AND CAN YOU DO SOMETHING WITH THE TANGLES?

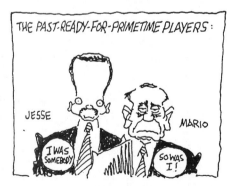

THE PAST-READY-FOR-PRIMETIME PLAYERS:

JESSE

I WAS SOMEBODY

MARIO

SO WAS I!

CONVENTION SKETCHBOOK *CHICAGO '96...*

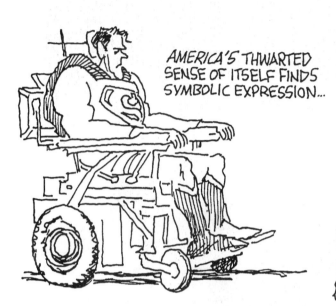

AMERICA'S THWARTED SENSE OF ITSELF FINDS SYMBOLIC EXPRESSION...

THE **DICK MORRIS** SCANDAL ROCKS THE CONVENTION:

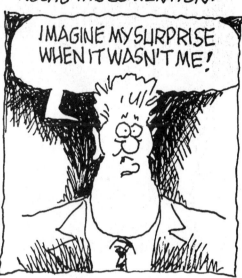

IMAGINE MY SURPRISE WHEN IT WASN'T ME!

THERE'S SOMETHING POETIC ABOUT CARL SANDBERG'S "CITY OF THE BROAD SHOULDERS" HOSTING BILL CLINTON'S PARTY

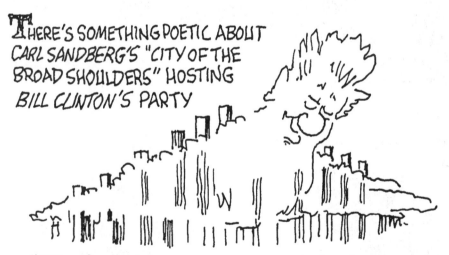

"The fog comes on little cat feet It sits looking

Over harbor and city on silent haunches and then moves on."

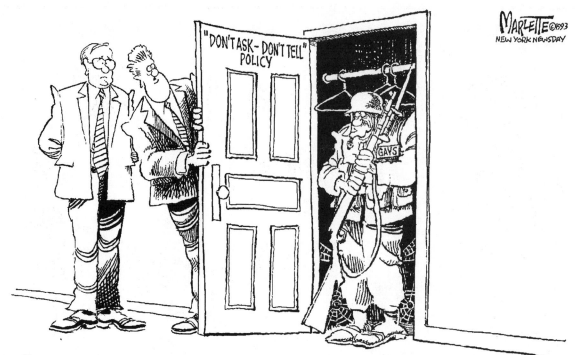

"OLD SOLDIERS NEVER DIE, BUT MAYBE HE'LL JUST FADE AWAY !..."

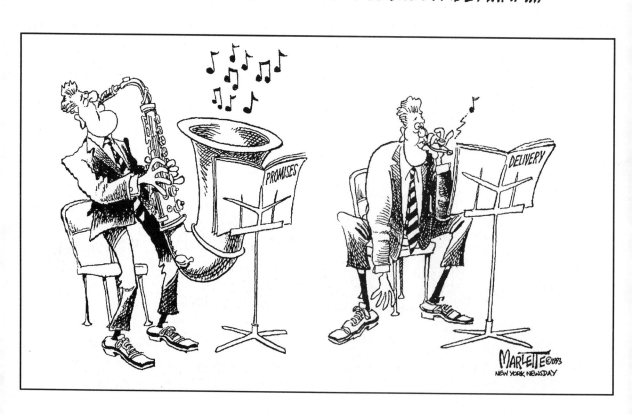

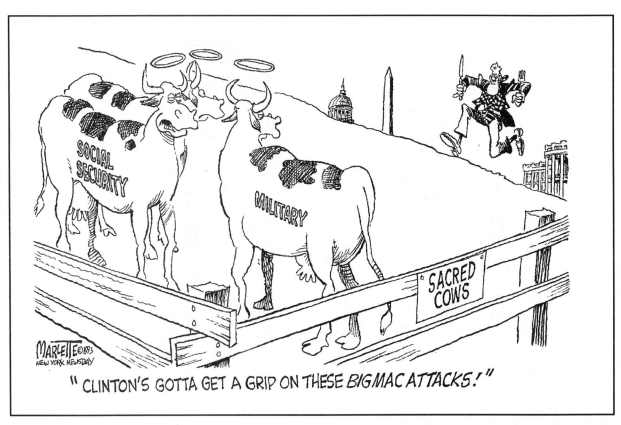

"CLINTON'S GOTTA GET A GRIP ON THESE *BIG MAC ATTACKS!*"

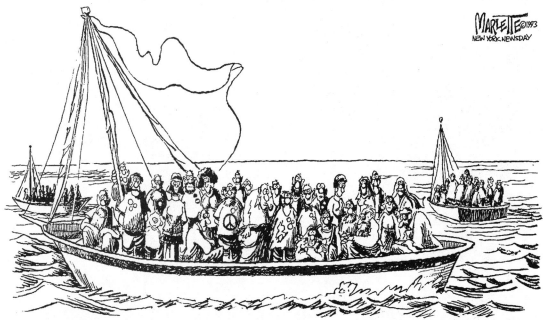

BOATLOADS OF *LIBERALS,* ADRIFT FOR YEARS AS POLITICAL REFUGEES, WERE INTERCEPTED BY THE COAST GUARD TODAY AS THEY MADE THEIR WAY UP THE POTOMAC SEEKING ASYLUM IN *BILL CLINTON'S AMERICA...*

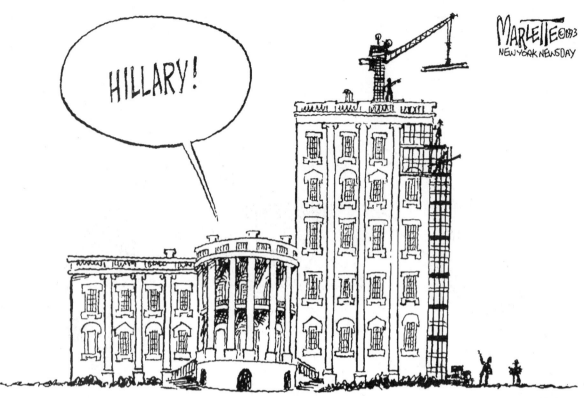

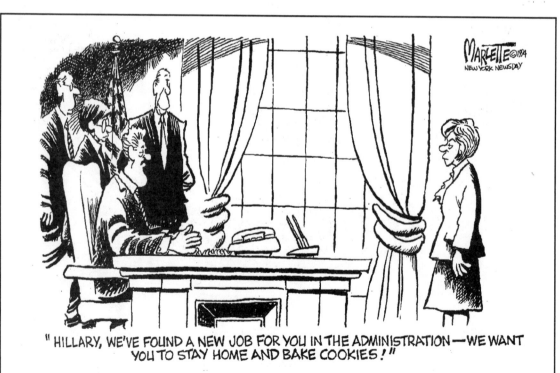

"HILLARY, WE'VE FOUND A NEW JOB FOR YOU IN THE ADMINISTRATION—WE WANT YOU TO STAY HOME AND BAKE COOKIES!"

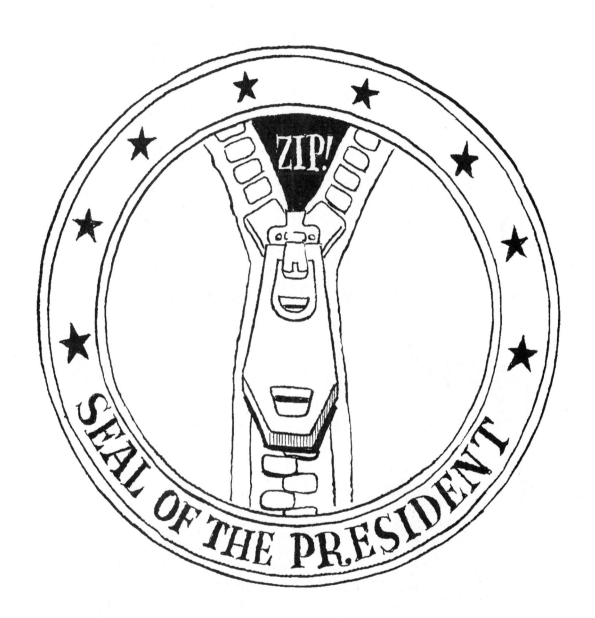

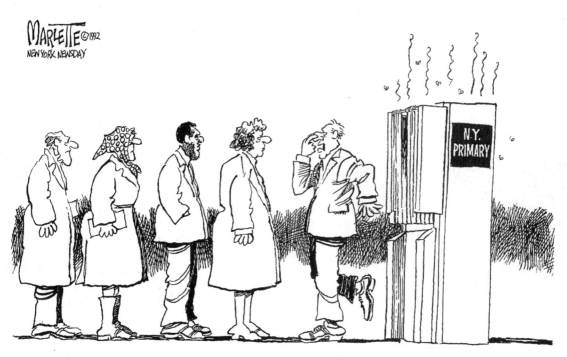

"I VOTED FOR CLINTON, BUT I DIDN'T INHALE!"

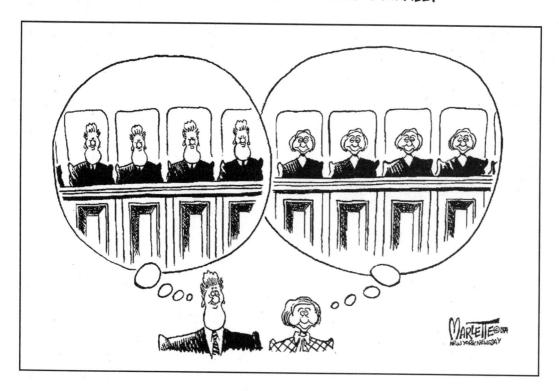

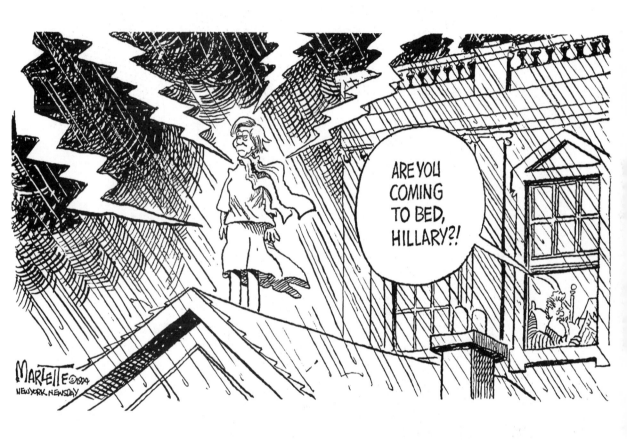

19

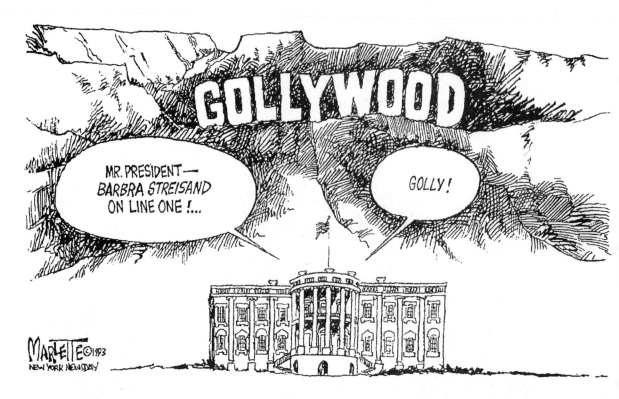

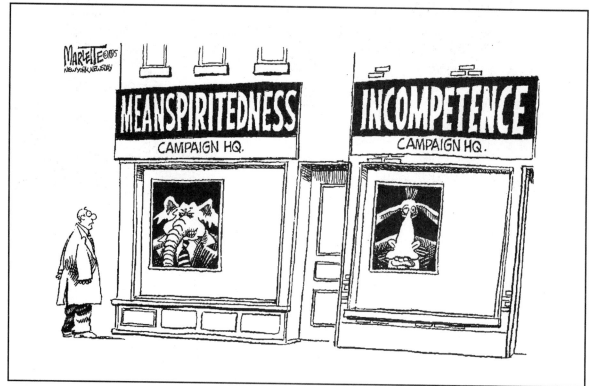

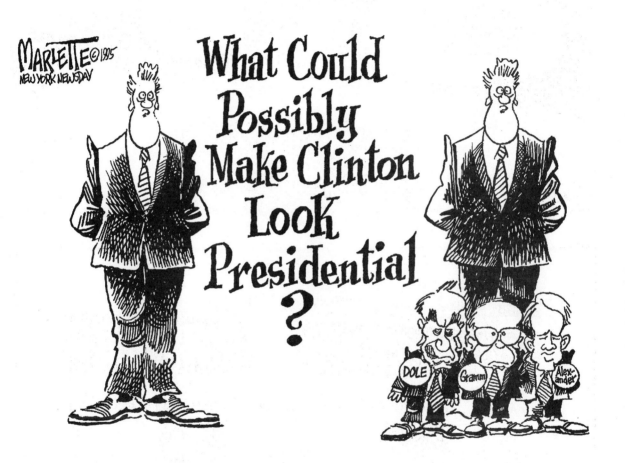

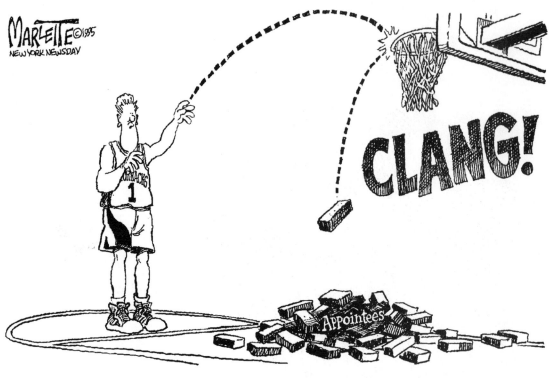

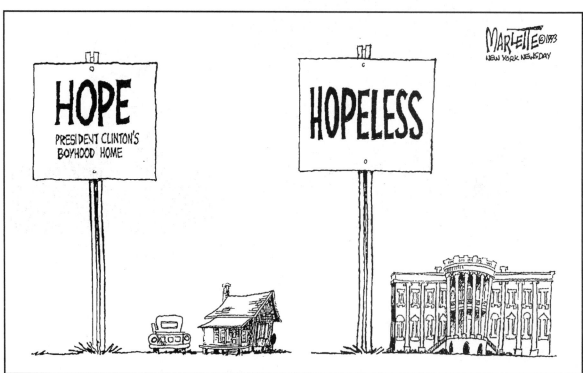

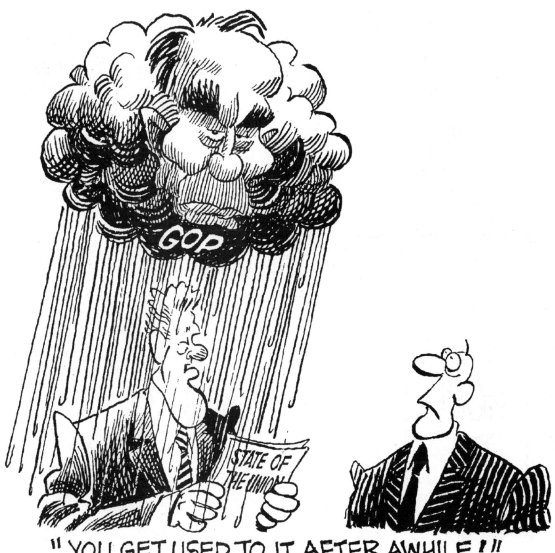

"YOU GET USED TO IT AFTER AWHILE!"

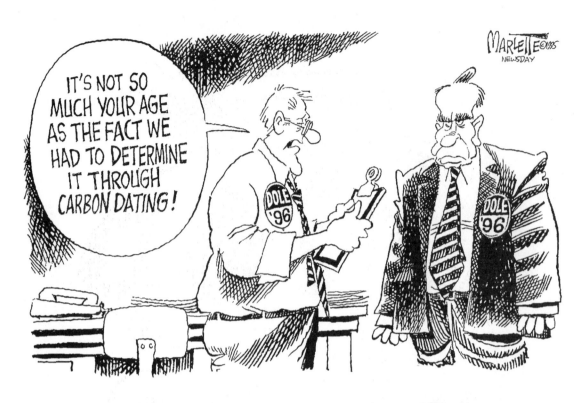

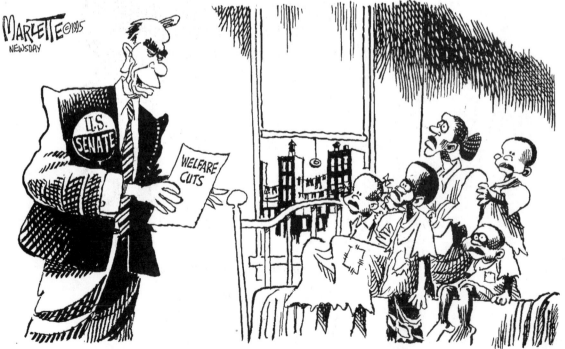

"JUST THINK OF IT AS DOWNSIZING!"

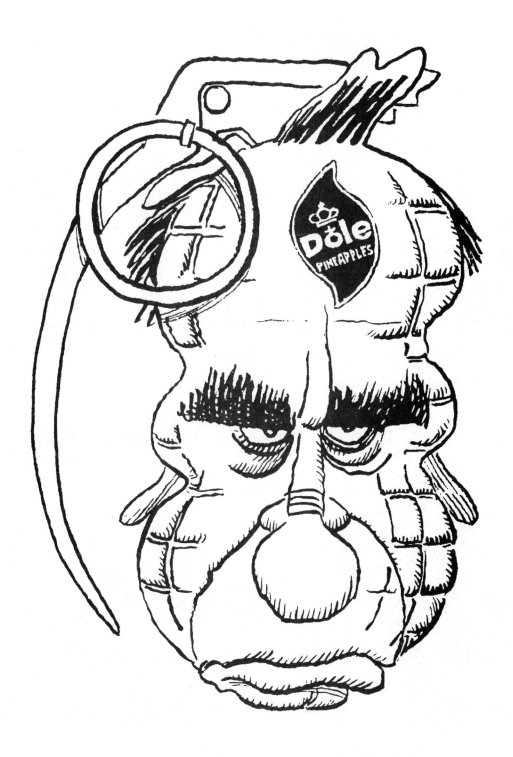

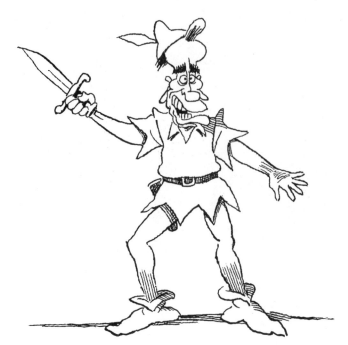

"JUST CLOSE YOUR EYES, THINK HAPPY THOUGHTS, AND FLY WITH ME TO NEVERLAND WHERE TAXES ARE LOWER AND BUDGETS ARE BALANCED!"

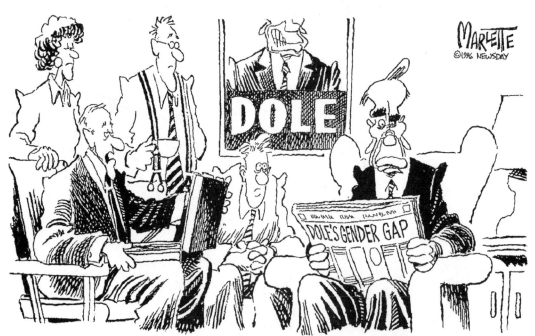

"WELL, FIRST YOU'RE GOING TO HAVE TO STOP CALLING IT THE 'BABE SITUATION'!"

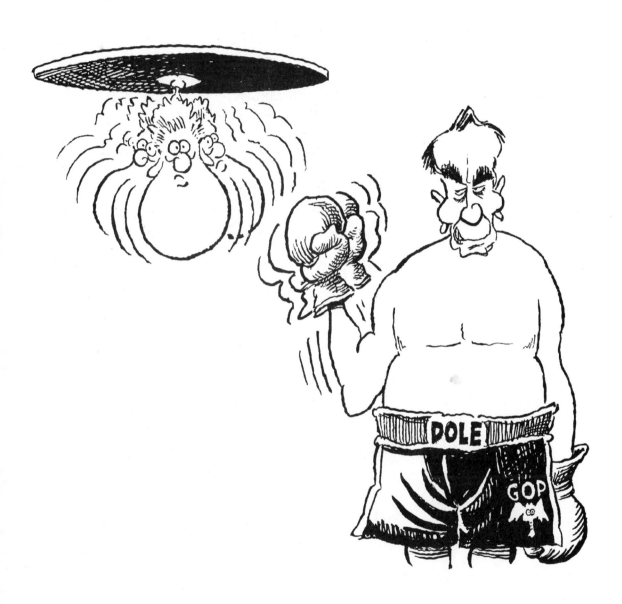

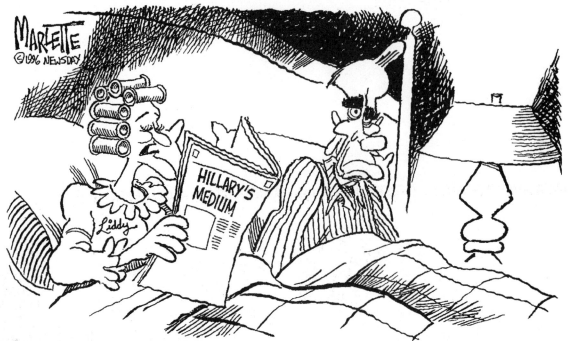

"BIG DEAL — I COMMUNE WITH THE DEAD ALL THE TIME!"

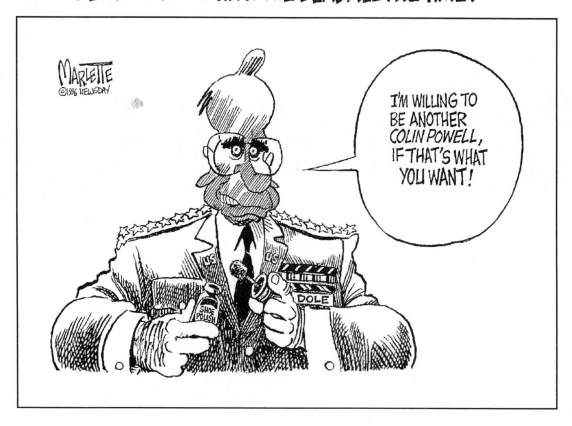

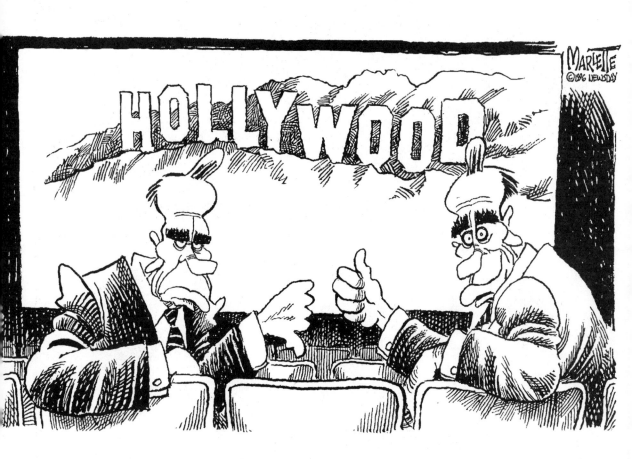

29

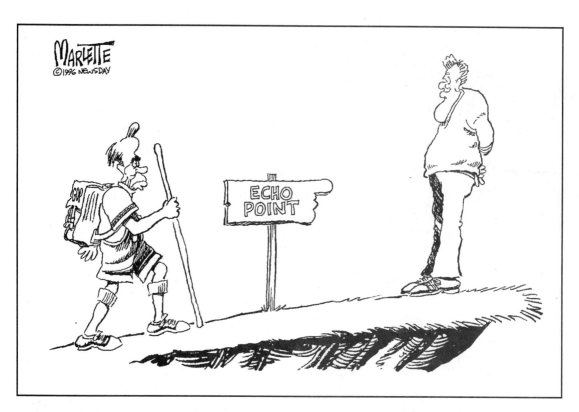

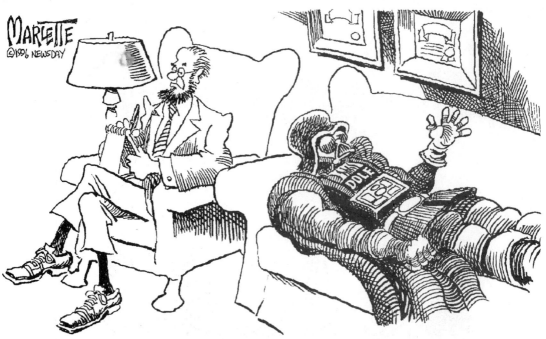

"I DON'T UNDERSTAND WHY PEOPLE DON'T WARM UP TO ME!"

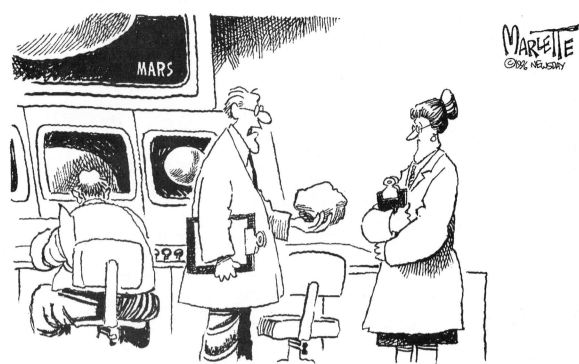

"—BUT WE STILL CAN'T FIND SIGNS OF LIFE IN THE *DOLE CAMPAIGN.*"

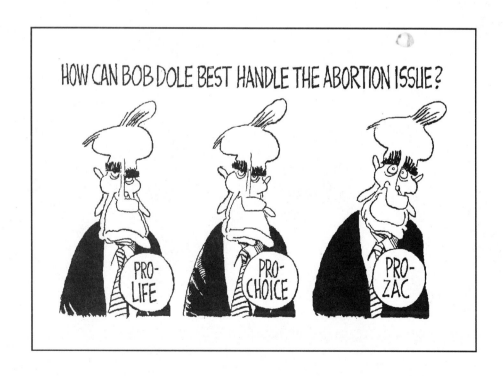

HOW CAN BOB DOLE BEST HANDLE THE ABORTION ISSUE?

PRO-LIFE   PRO-CHOICE   PRO-ZAC

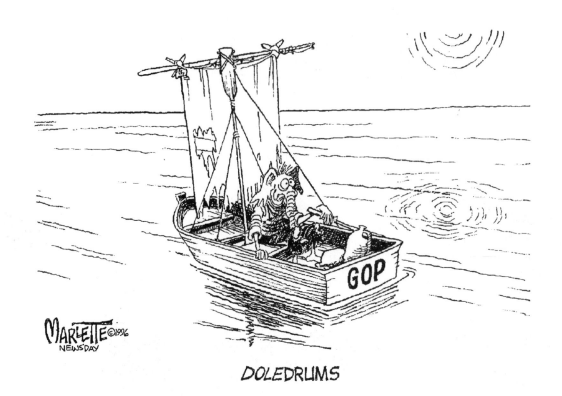

DOLEDRUMS

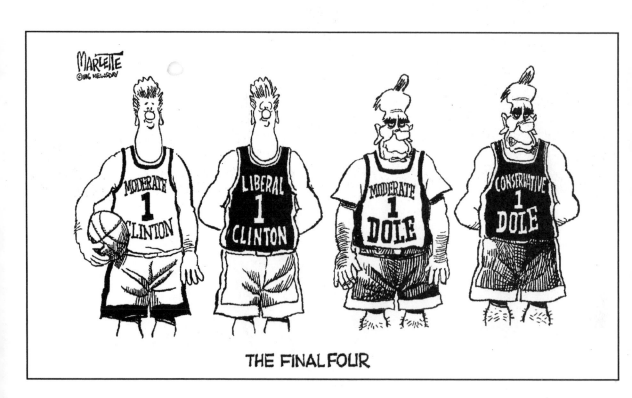

THE FINAL FOUR

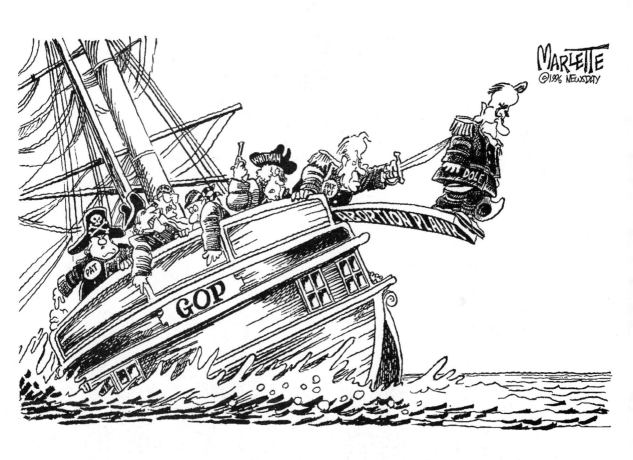

33

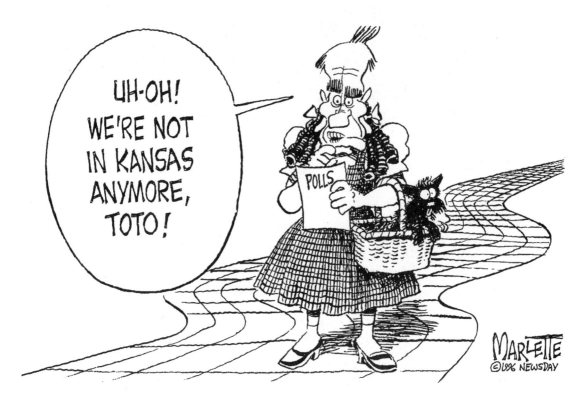

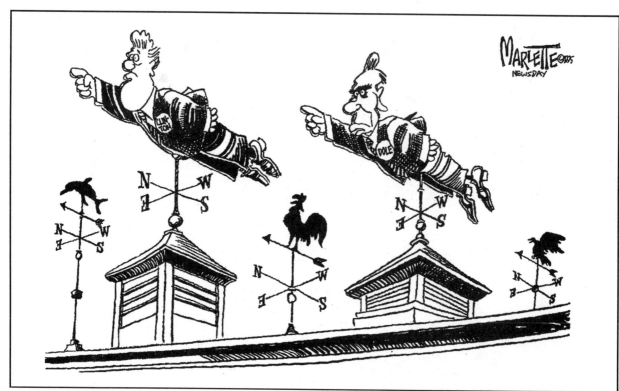

How I Got a Cartoon Idea

I like cartoon ideas that are natural—unforced, spontaneous and direct, the kind the reader gets instantly, because the artist has done all the work. Nothing has to be deciphered or figured out. Nobody has to think, "Oh. I see what he's driving at." There is no distance, no gap between the original impulse, that electrical charge of wit or insight, that leap of the synapses called inspiration, and what shows up on paper. It is as if the artist's neurons are firing directly onto the drawing paper, like his ink supply flows straight from his carotid artery. These kinds of ideas are up from the cellars, out of the depths, instinctive, and surprising. They come as a result of a highly-developed capacity for free association combined with a killer instinct.

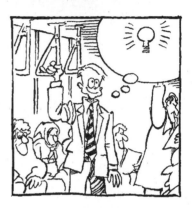

After settling on a topic, I get cartoon ideas by sketching and thinking, doodling and noodling. When the California Supreme Court ruled against affirmative action I wanted to comment on it. Here is a rough rehash of the kind of chaotic thinking process that led to a cartoon.

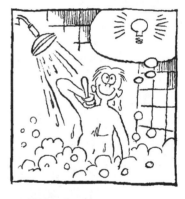

I begin by thinking about affirmative action, reverse discrimination . . . The fact that the ruling came from California's university system makes me think of racism in California, which leads me to think of the famous video images of the LAPD beating

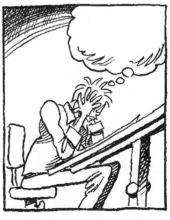

35

up Rodney King, which prompts sketches of a figure labeled California Supreme Court beating up lady justice . . . Or maybe Mark Fuhrman beating up . . . uh . . . Mark Fuhrman . . . Hold on . . . Start over . . . Let's see now . . . Reverse discrimination in California . . . What is that like? . . . Hmmm . . . Come to think of it, you never heard Ray Charles do a cover of a Beach Boys tune! I try to remember the lyrics of "Help Me, Rhonda," which reminds me of Kato Kaelin and how he kind of looks like one of the Beach Boys . . . Maybe Dennis Wilson on Prozac. But wait—I'm getting off track. I keep drifting to the O.J. trial . . . Let's see . . . What do we have here? . . . Angry White Guys in California . . . First, I think of Bobby Hurley drafted by the Sacramento Kings . . . L.A. Kings, Wayne Gretzky . . . No . . . Angry Middle-Aged White Guys . . . Hmmm . . . Barry Diller, David Geffen, Katzenberg, Spielberg, Mike Ovitz, and ten thousand short, Armani-suited CAA agents in Tai Chi stances . . . Wrong way. Dead End . . . Hmmm . . . Angry white guys, angry white guys, ulcers, Pepto Bismol, high blood pressure, clogged arteries, florid faces, Michael Douglas, Kirk Douglas, Douglas MacArthur, MacArthur Foundation, Genius grants, Foster Grants . . . No, I'm getting away from it again . . . White and Colored water fountains . . . White and Colored entrances . . . White guys singing, "We Shall Overcome" . . . We Shall Overkill . . . We shall Overcompensate . . . Naaa . . . Discrimination . . . We Reserve the Right to Refuse Service to Anyone . . . White Men Can't Jump . . . White Men Can't Jumpstart Their Careers . . . Wait . . . Let's start over . . . Why do privileged white guys feel victimized? What kind of jobs do whites feel that blacks have taken from them? Good question . . . Power Forward for the Houston Rockets? Vice President for Vertical Affairs? Band leader for The Tonight Show? African American studies professor at Berkeley? NFL running back? Blind blues singer? Vice President for Blind Blues Operations? . . . Wait. I'm onto something. What kind of jobs do angry whites feel would be okay to give minorities first dibs on? Porters, housekeepers, chauffeurs, bussing tables, shoeshine stands . . .

Shoeshine stands! Now that's a classic image . . . There's got to be something there! . . . An angry white guy getting a shoeshine by a black guy at a shoeshine stand! I bet some whites would even feel cheated out of traditional reacially stereotyped jobs . . . Hey! So why not show that?! Bingo! The caption wrote itself.

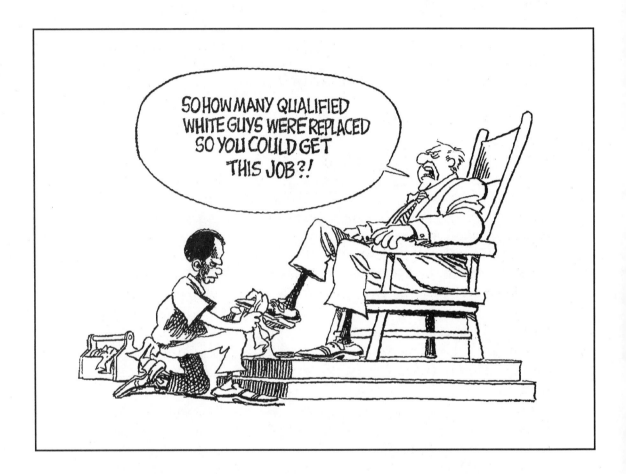

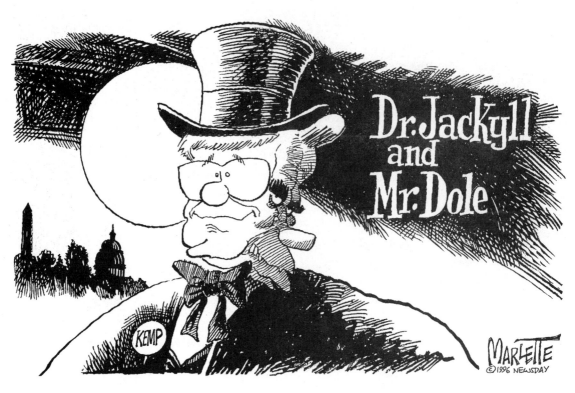

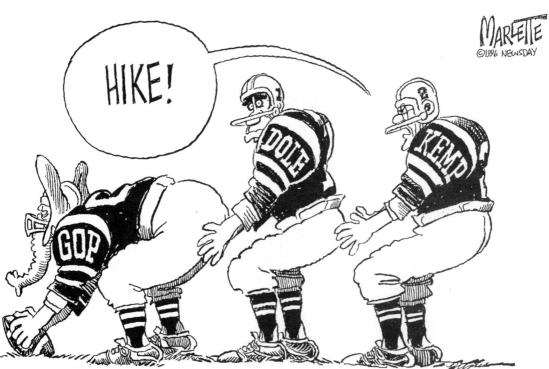

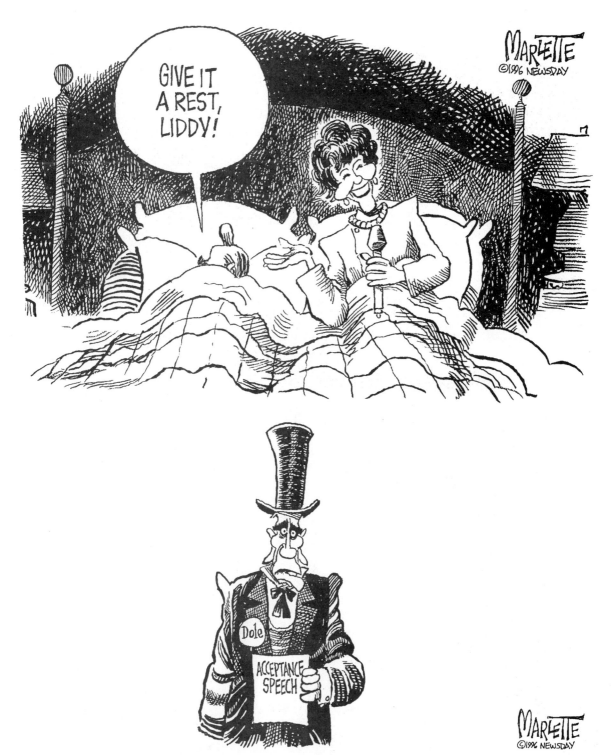

INFRARED PHOTO OF *PAT BUCHANAN* ILLEGALLY CROSSING BORDER TO SNEAK INTO GOP CONVENTION

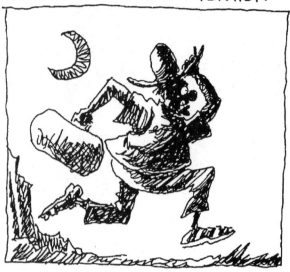

SHOCKING SAME-PARTY MARRIAGE

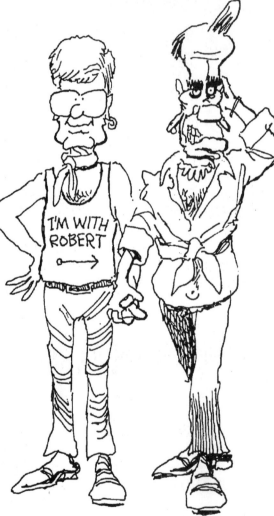

THE PARTY'S MEANNESS OF SPIRIT WENT UNDER COVER DURING PRIMETIME...

DOWN, NEWT!

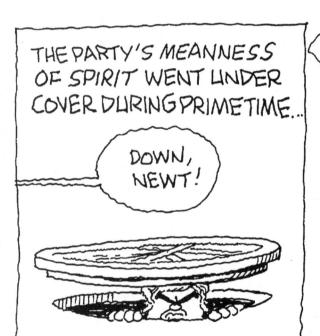

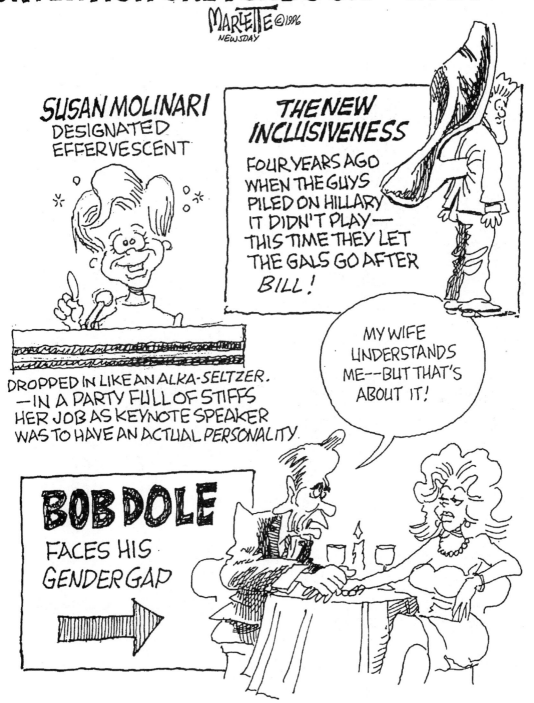

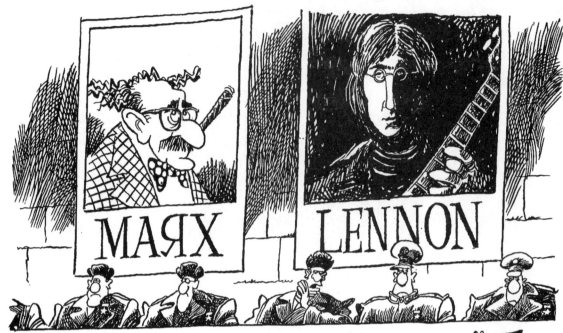

"GORBACHEV'S GOING TOO FAST!"

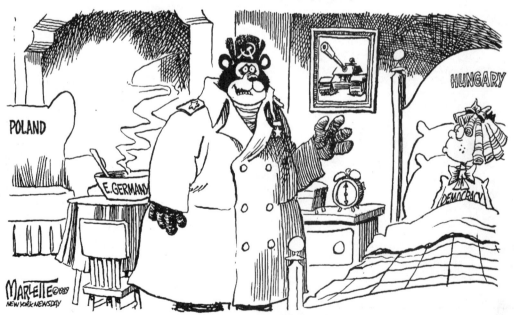

"SOMEONE'S BEEN SITTING IN MY CHAIR, EATING MY PORRIDGE AND SLEEPING
IN MY BED, BUT HEY— I CAN LIVE WITH THAT!"

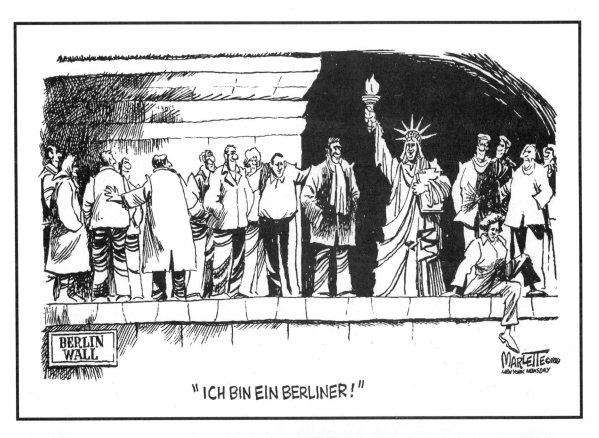

"ICH BIN EIN BERLINER!"

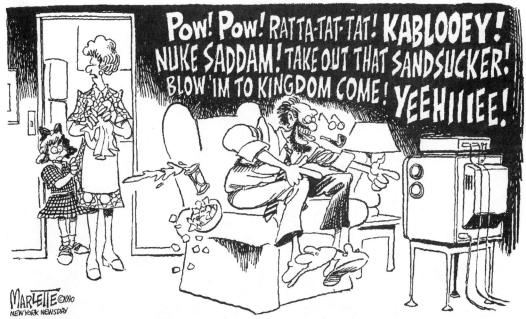

"YOUR FATHER'S A BABY-BOOM LIBERAL, DEAR—HE'S NEVER HAD A WAR HE COULD SUPPORT BEFORE!"

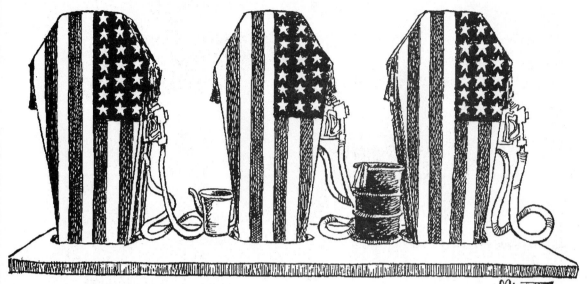

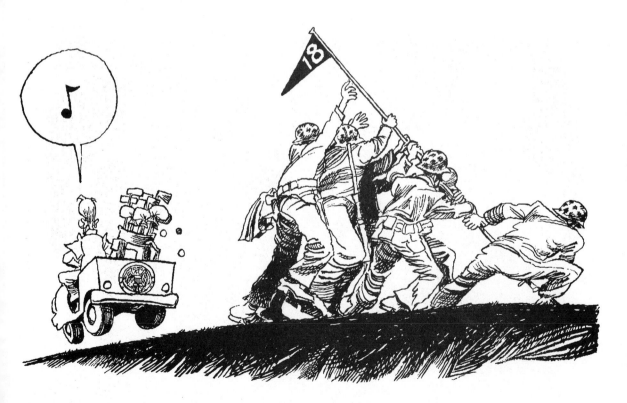

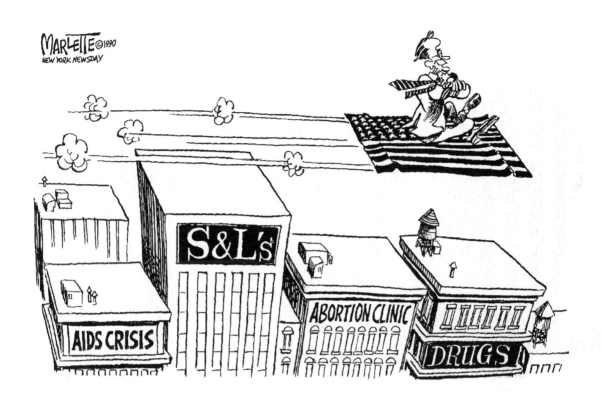

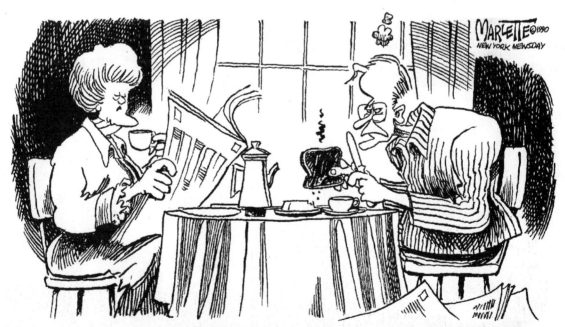

"NO, GEORGE — WE DON'T NEED A CONSTITUTIONAL AMENDMENT AGAINST BURNING THE *TOAST!*"

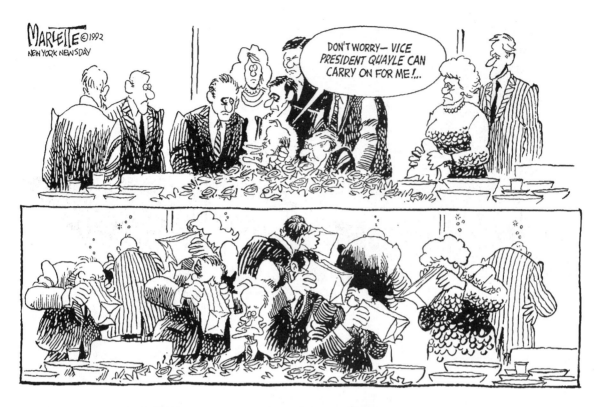

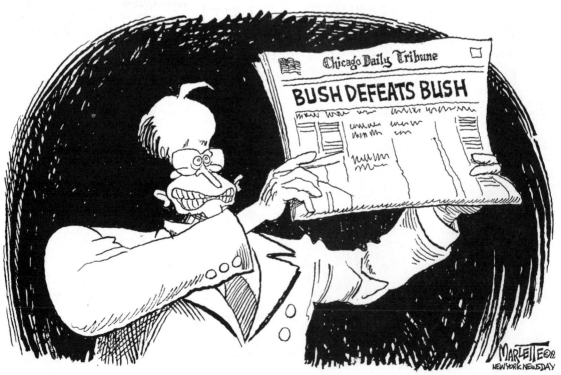

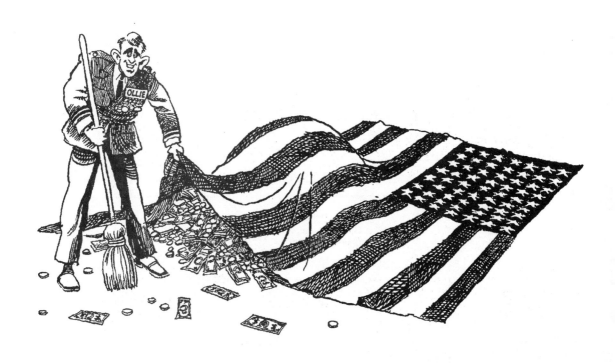

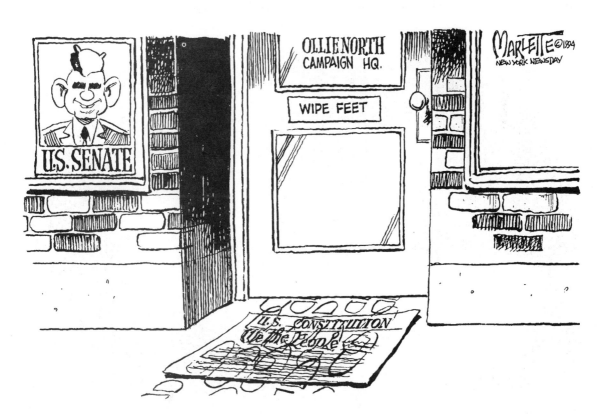

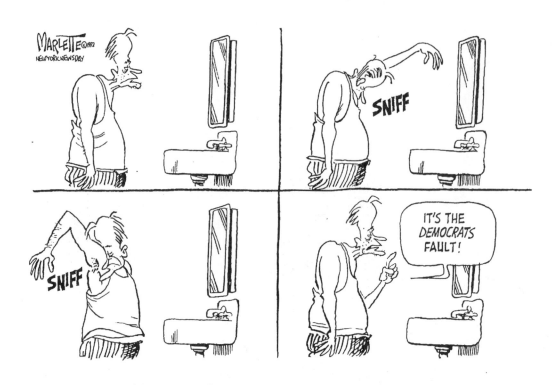

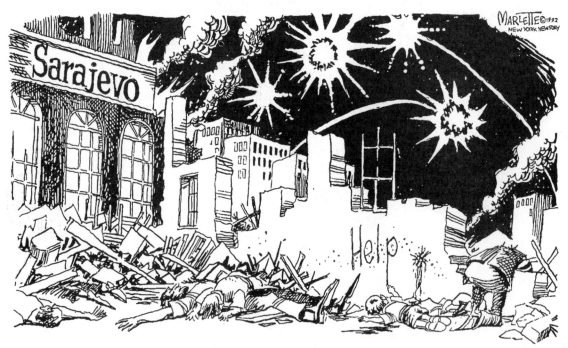

Gave Proof Through The Night That No Oil Is Drilled There...

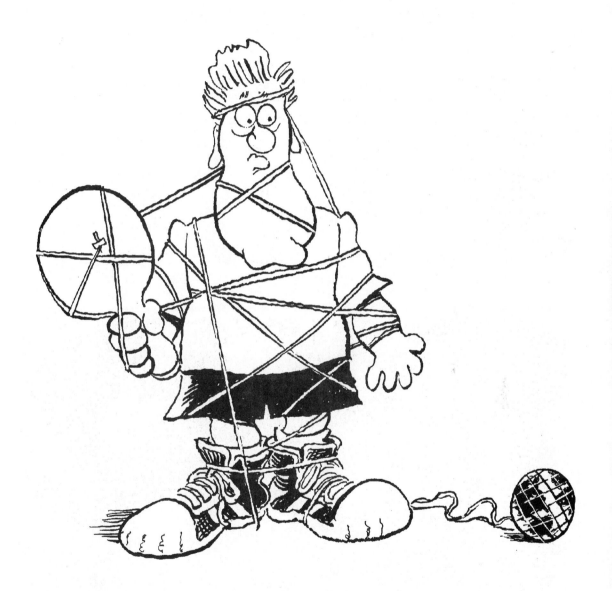

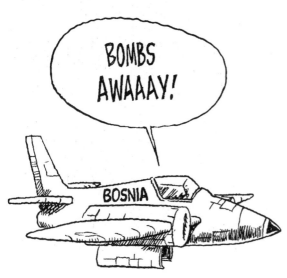

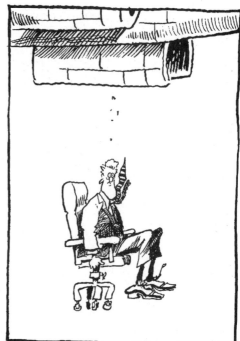

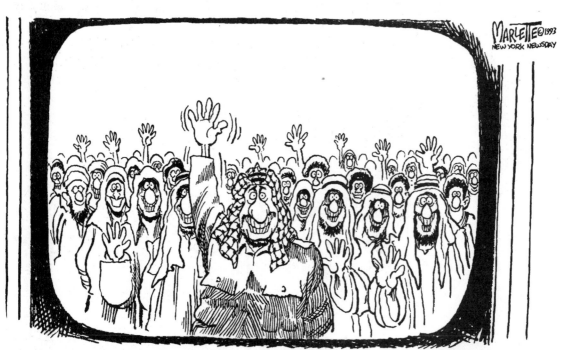

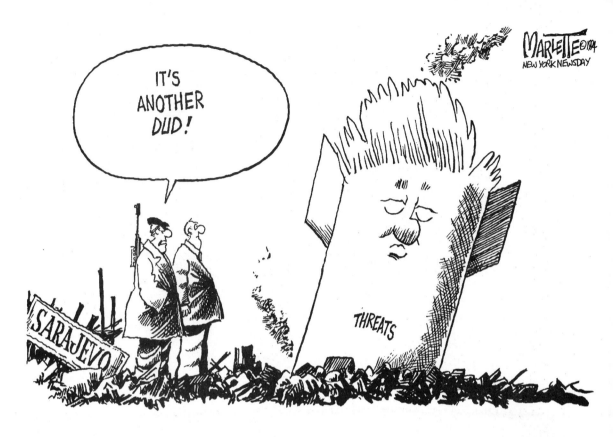

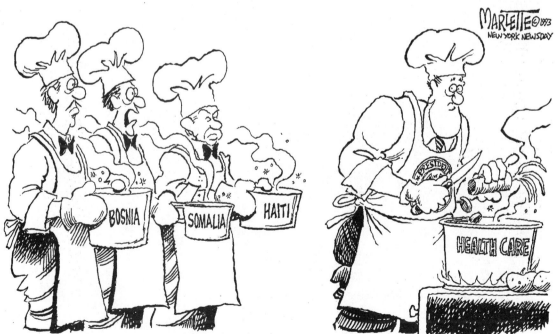

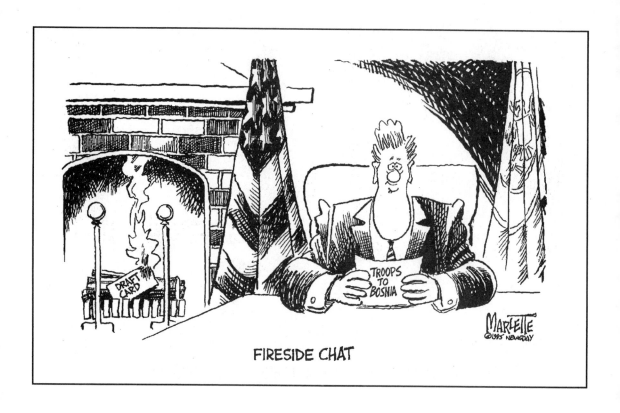

FIRESIDE CHAT

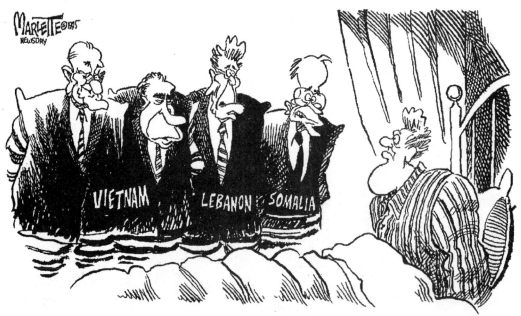

"WE ARE THE GHOSTS OF *CHRISTMAS PAST!*"

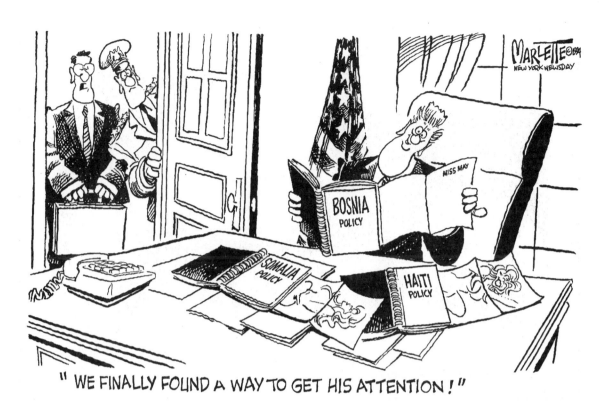

" WE FINALLY FOUND A WAY TO GET HIS ATTENTION ! "

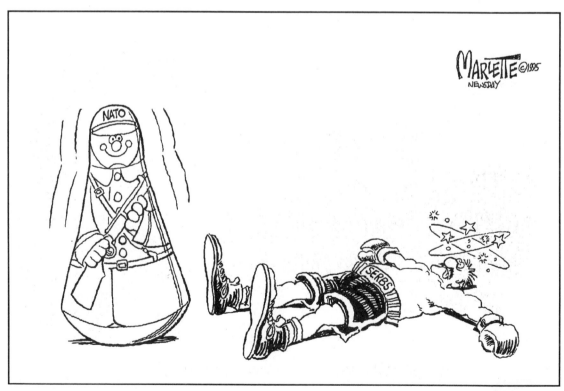

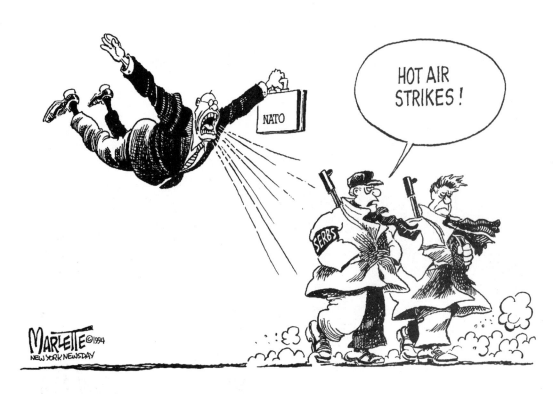

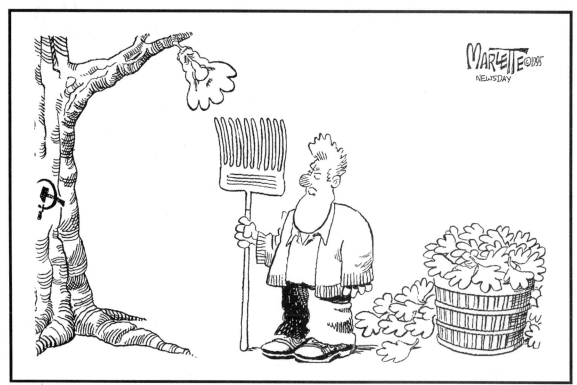

54

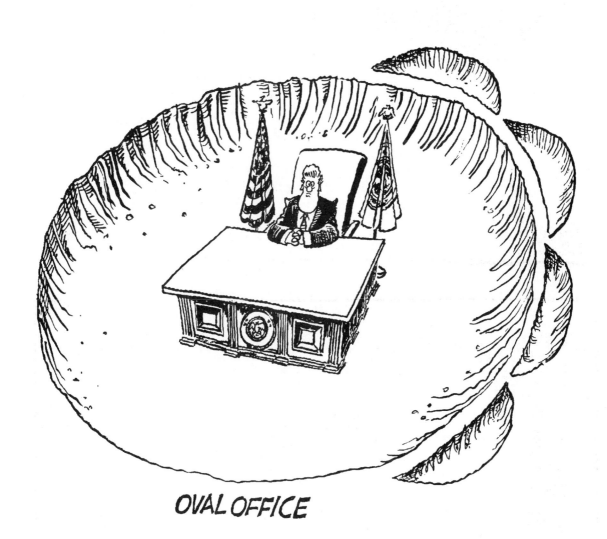

OVAL OFFICE

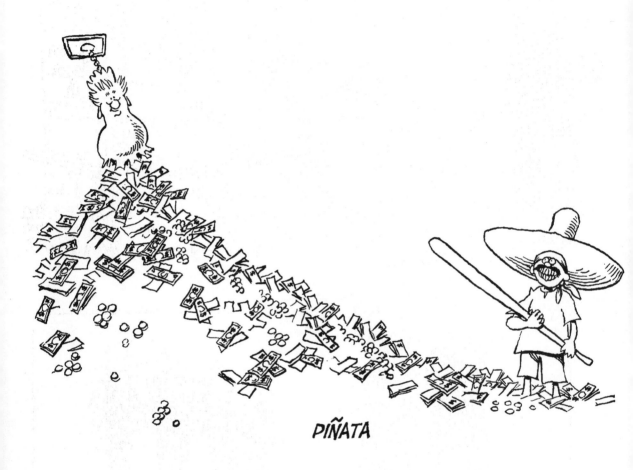

PIÑATA

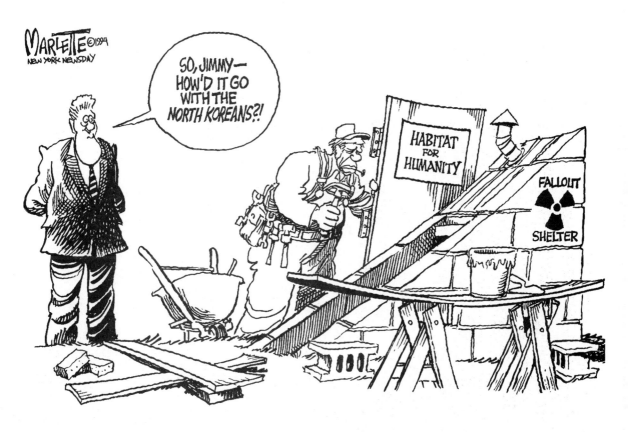

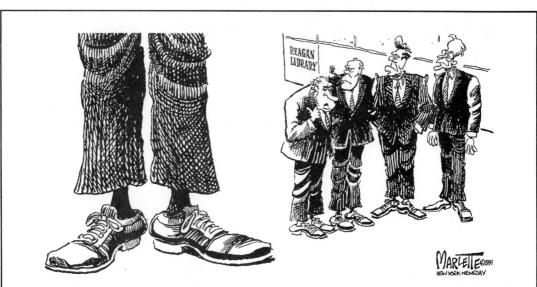

"SOMEBODY EXPLAIN TO CARTER THAT YOU'RE SUPPOSED TO GROW IN OFFICE AND THEN, DAMMIT, *KNOCK IT OFF!*"

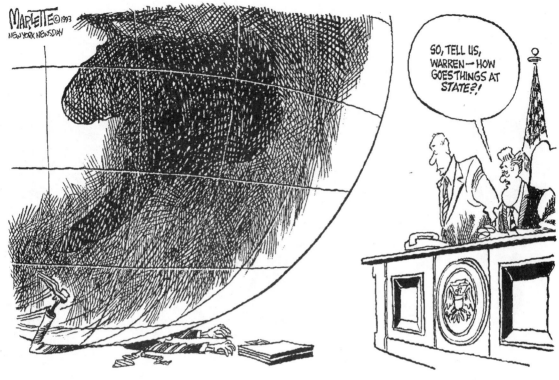

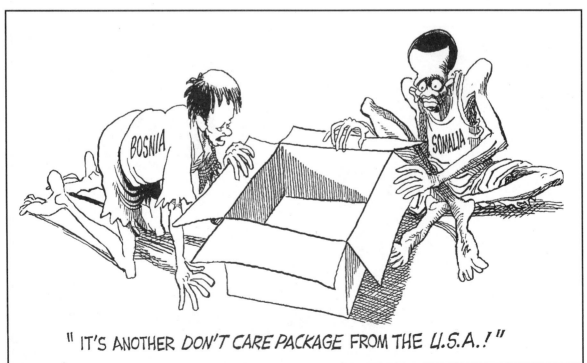

" IT'S ANOTHER *DON'T CARE PACKAGE* FROM THE *U.S.A.!* "

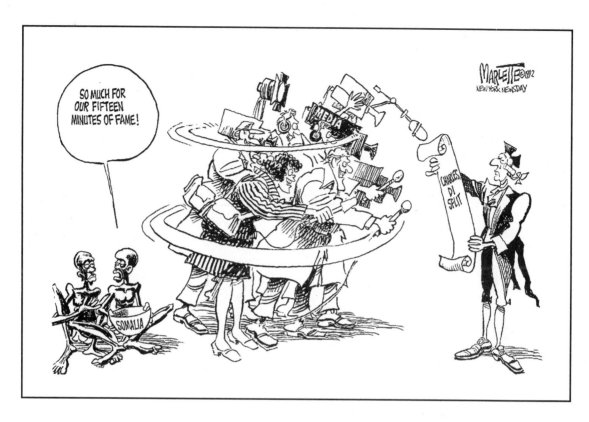

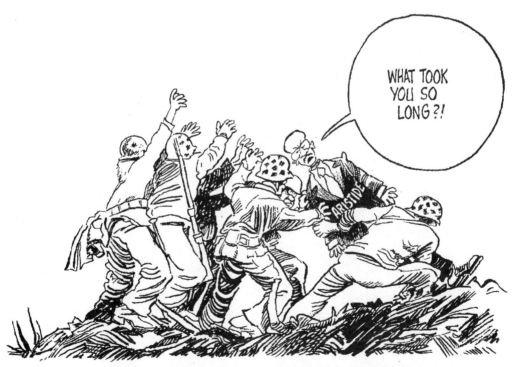

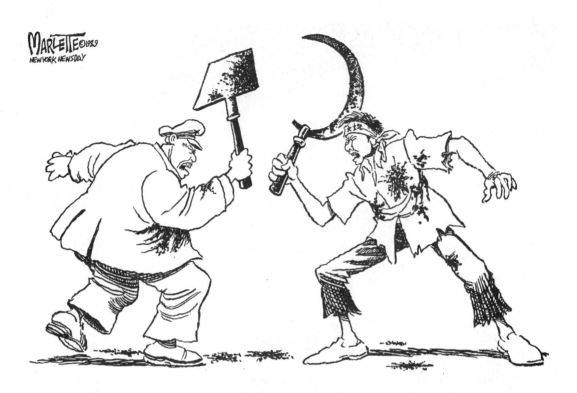

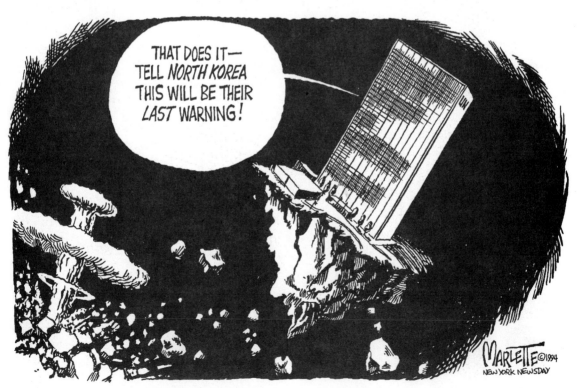

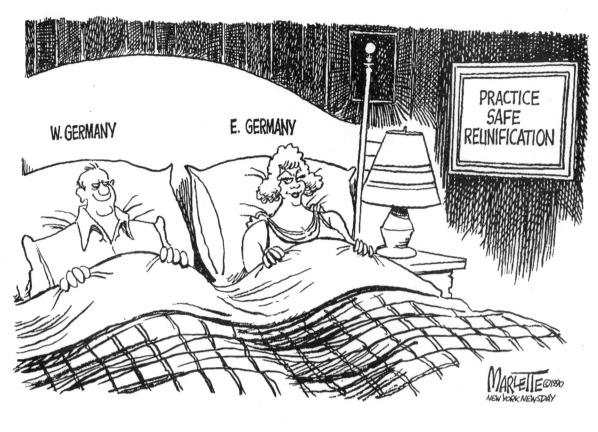

W. GERMANY   E. GERMANY

PRACTICE SAFE REUNIFICATION

MARLETTE ©1990
NEW YORK NEWSDAY

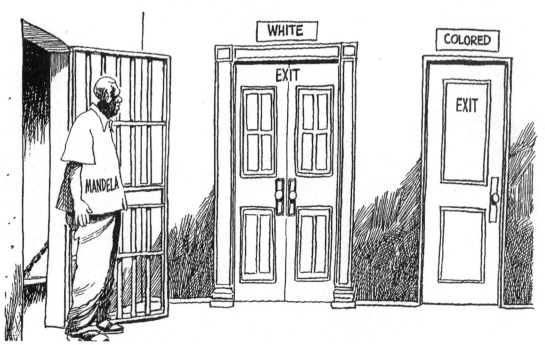

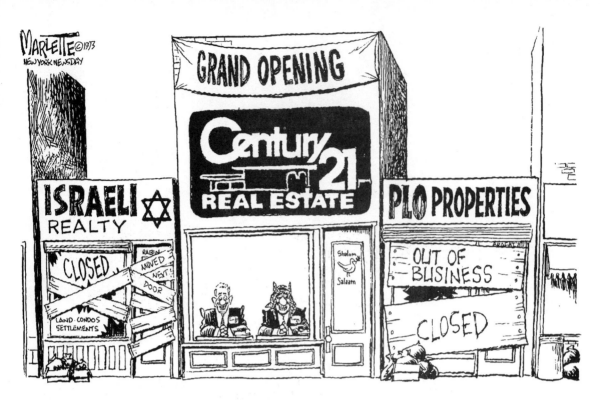

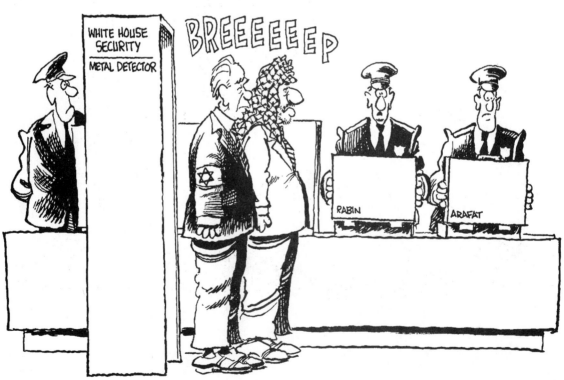

"PLOWSHARES!"

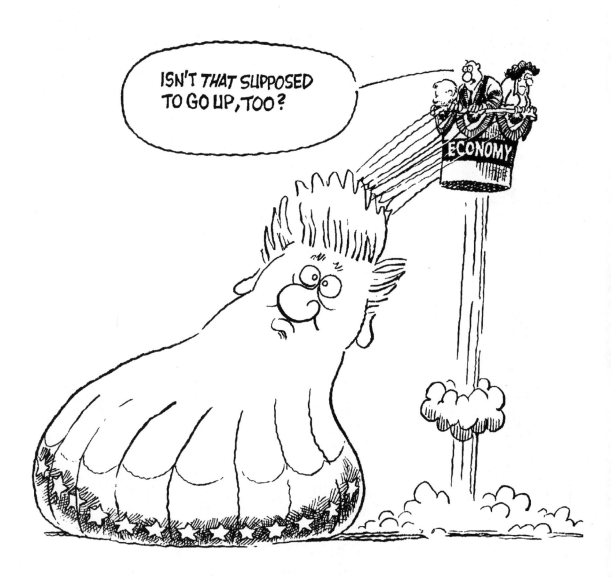

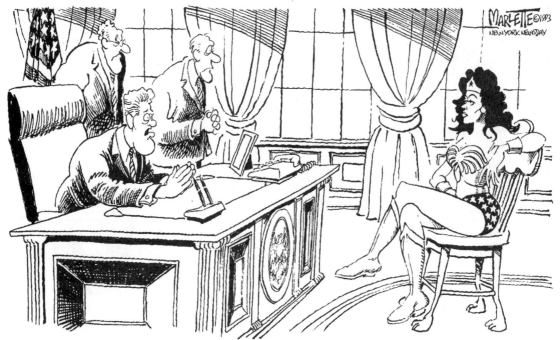

"NEVER MIND YOUR LAW ENFORCEMENT EXPERIENCE — DID YOU EVER HIRE AN *ILLEGAL ALIEN ?!...*"

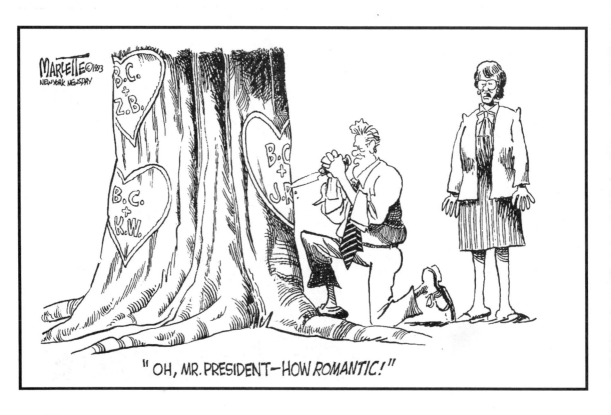

" OH, MR. PRESIDENT—HOW *ROMANTIC !*"

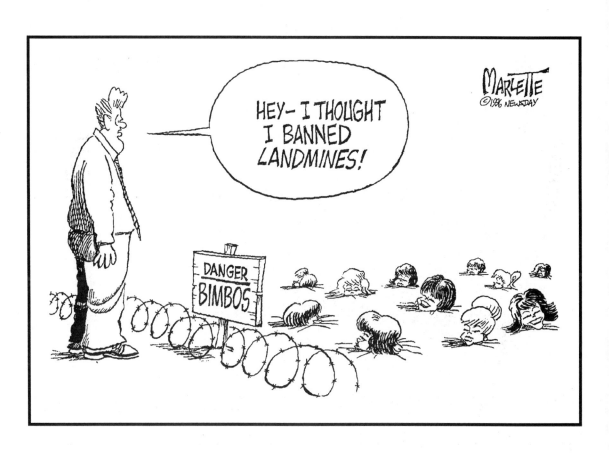

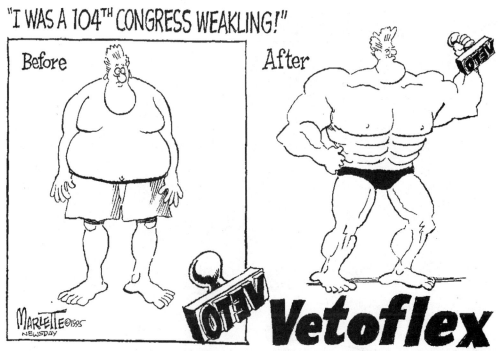

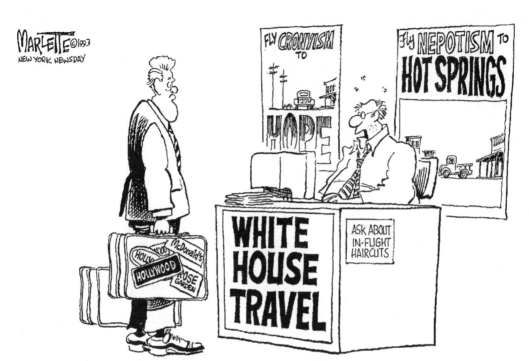

" WE GOT A SPECIAL ON ONE-WAY TICKETS TO LITTLE ROCK !... "

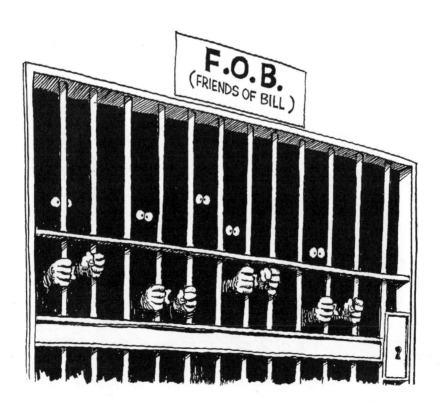

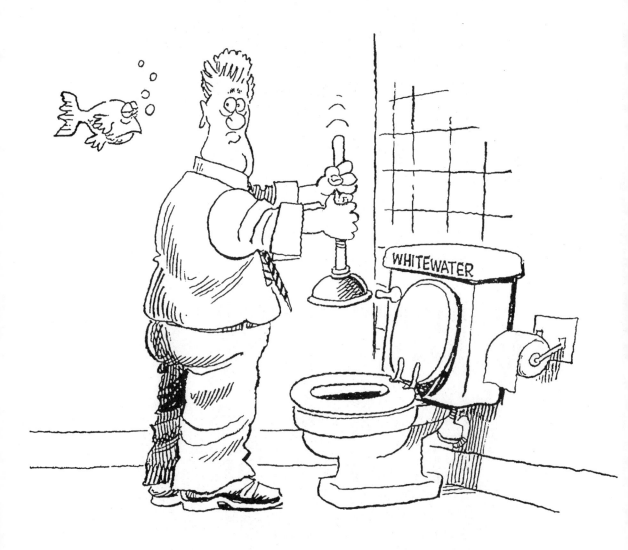

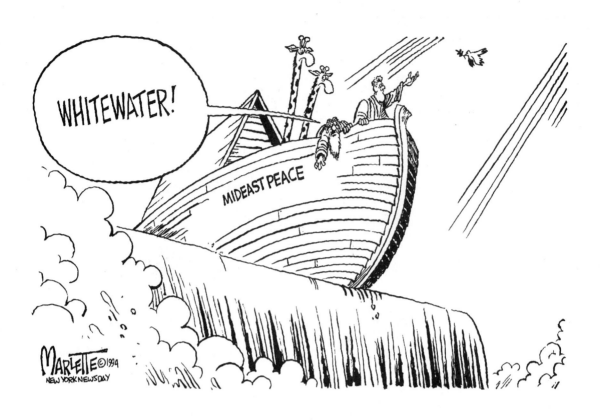

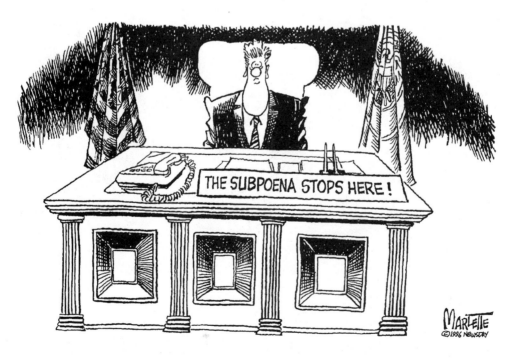

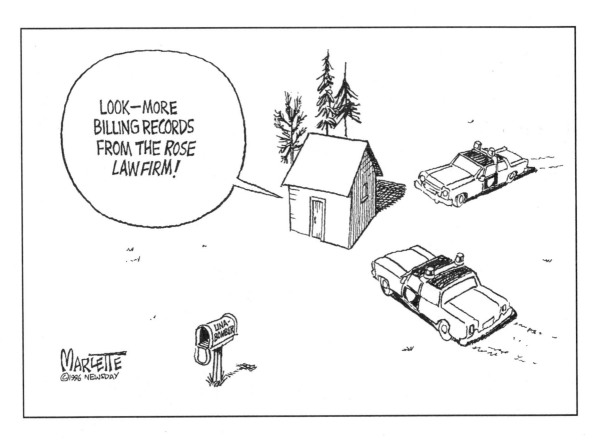

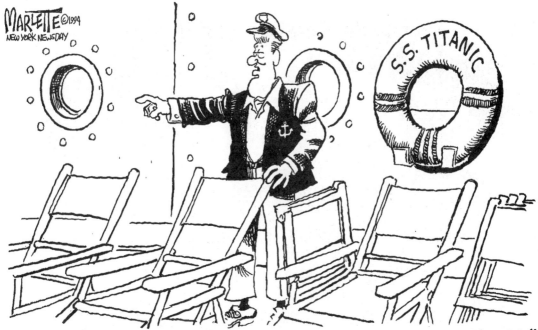

"PANETTA! YOU SIT HERE!.... McLARTY OVER THERE!...I'M REARRANGING THE DECK CHAIRS!..."

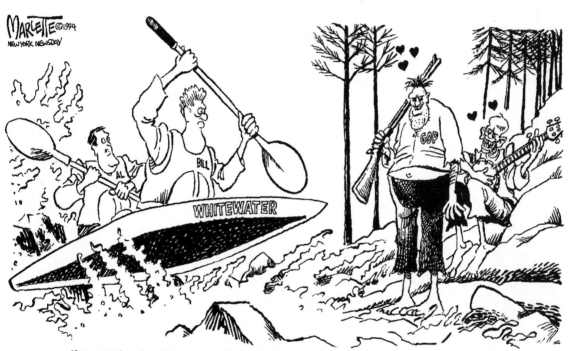

"SAY, WASN'T IT SOMEWHERE ALONG ABOUT HERE THEY SHOT THE LOVE
SCENE FROM *DELIVERANCE* ?!..."

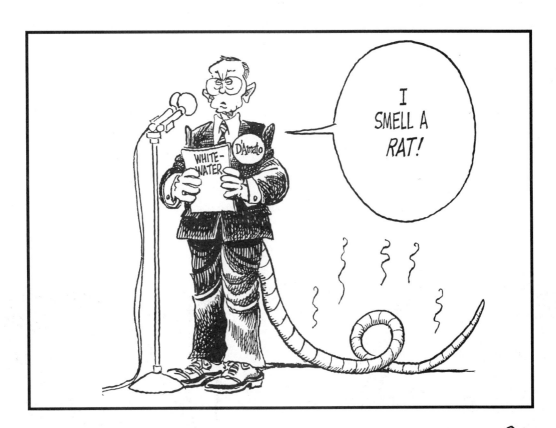

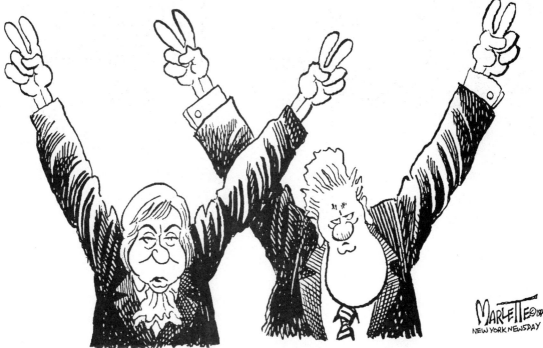

"WE ARE NOT A CROOK!"

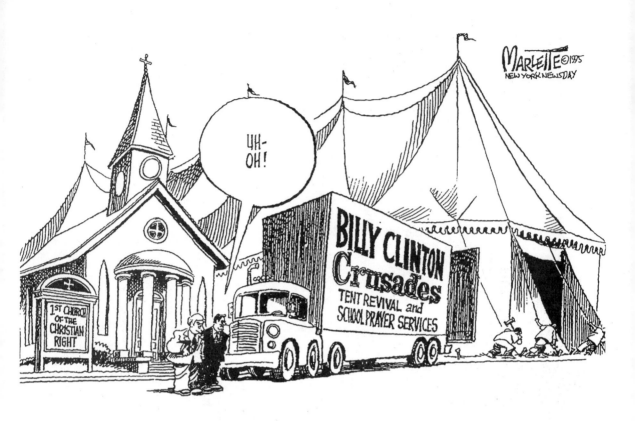

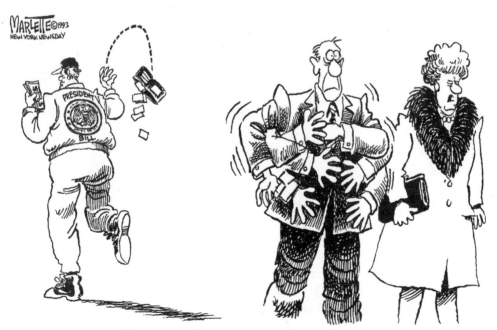

"SO THAT EXPLAINS THE *HUGGING.!...*"

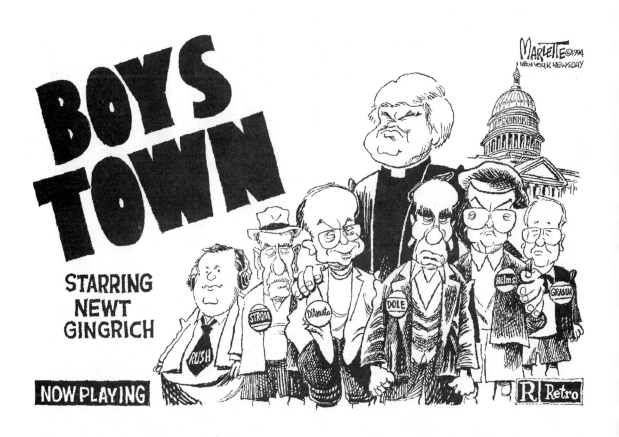

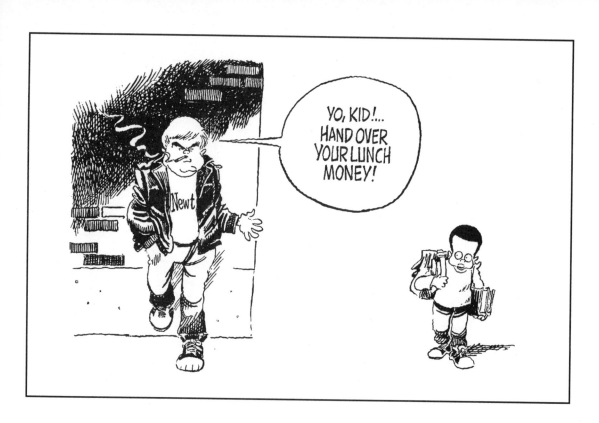

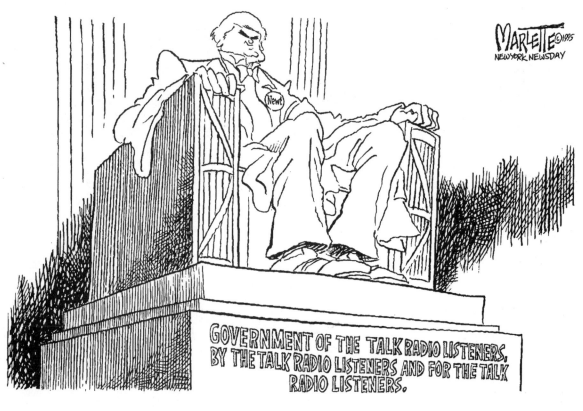

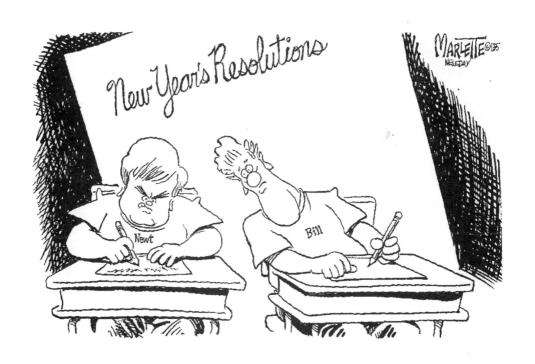

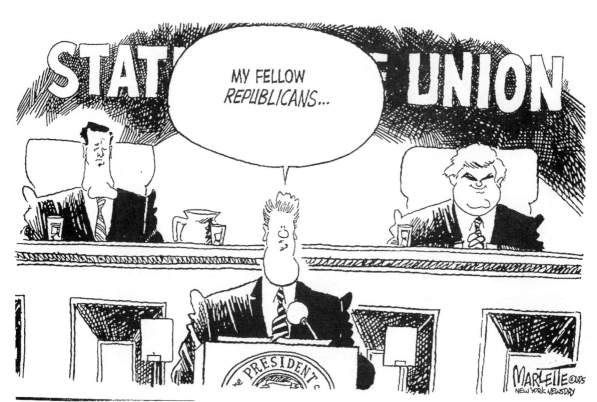

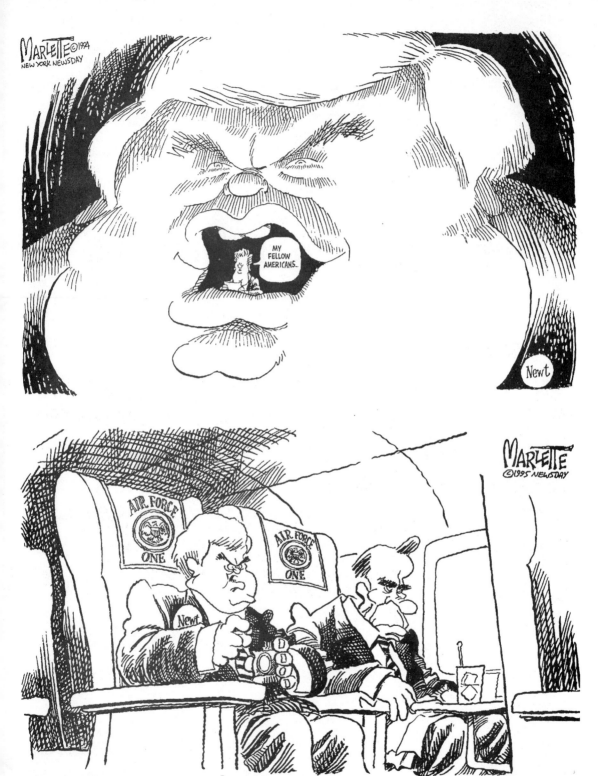

"WHAT—STALE PEANUTS?!...WELL, SO MUCH FOR AID TO DEPENDENT CHILDREN!"

The Branch Republicans

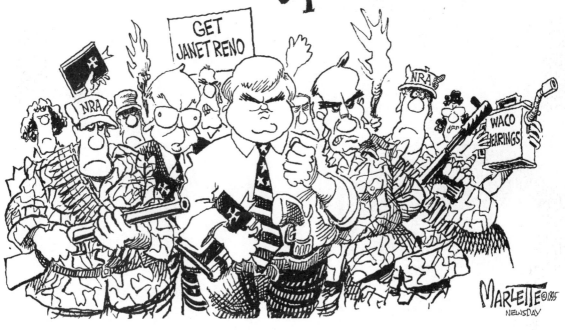

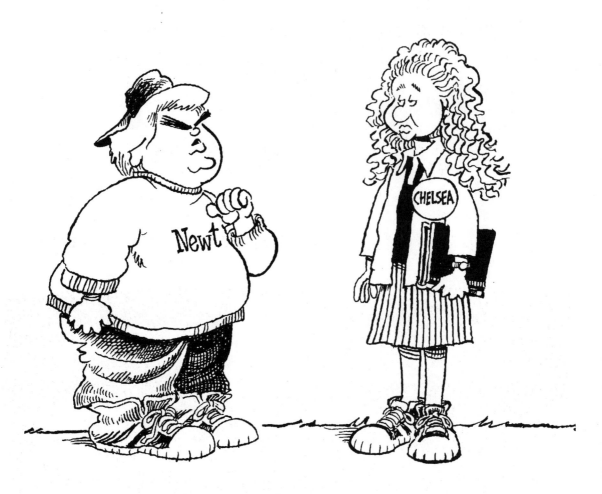

"MY MOM CAN BEAT UP YOUR MOM!"

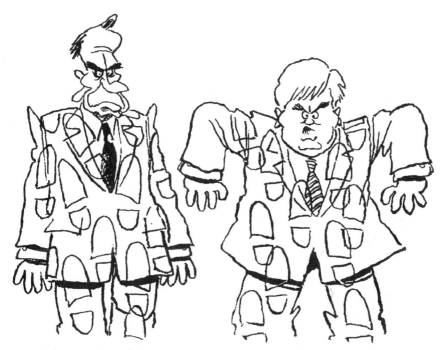

" I THOUGHT YOU SAID CLINTON DOESN'T WALK THE WALK!"

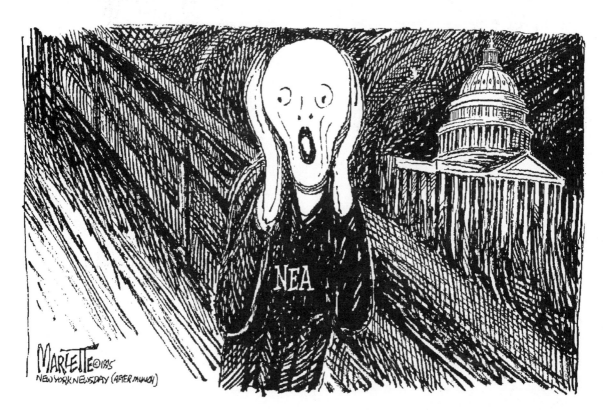

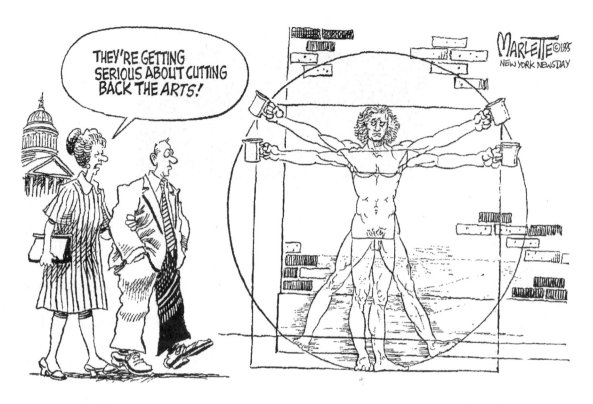

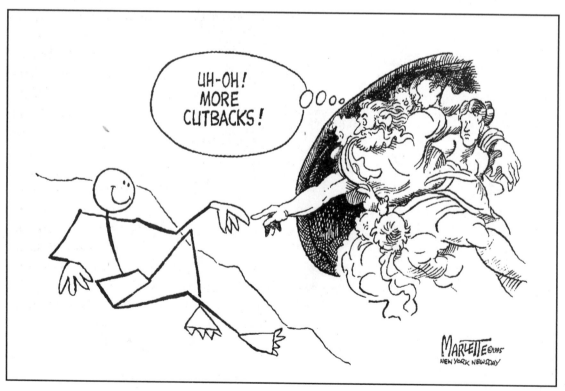

Helms in a Handbasket

From the New York Times, October 29, 1990

Doug Marlette's comic strip "Kudzu" often explores the clash between old values and modern life in the changing South, as represented by the mythical town of Bypass, N.C. Now, he is offering the view from Bypass of Senator Jesse Helms's campaign for re-election. But this is a subject of sensitivity in the real North Carolina.

Mr. Marlette, a native of the state who now works in New York for *Newsday*, produced a series of strips lampooning the Senator's struggle to come to grips with the end of the cold war.

"Nobody's out to get me," the Senator tells a psychiatrist in the strip, shortly before solving his problem by announcing a Senate hearing into the International Artistic Conspiracy, as well as a decision by the National Endowment for the Arts to suppress production of black velvet art.

As is often the case in politics, the line between reality and satire can blur. In "Kudzu," a mock Helms commercial attacks his opponent for holding fund-raising events "in places like New York and San Francisco, if you know what I mean." The real-life Helms campaign is using a television commercial saying that the Senator's opponent, Harvey Gantt, "has raised thousands of dollars in gay and lesbian bars in San Francisco, New York and Washington."

Some North Carolina newspapers got edgy. The Raleigh news and Observer suspended the comic strip until it stops lampooning Mr. Helms or until the election, whichever comes first. *The Charlotte Observer* and the *Winston-Salem Journal* moved the strip to the opinion pages.

81

FOR YEARS, SENATOR JESSE HELMS ALWAYS CHECKED UNDER HIS BED AT NIGHT FOR COMMIES...

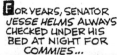

...UNTIL THE COLLAPSE OF WORLD COMMUNISM SENT THE SENATOR INTO A TAILSPIN...

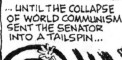
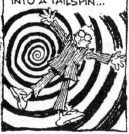

...WITHOUT THE COMFORTS OF COLD WAR CERTITUDE AND THE PLEASURES OF PARANOIA, HE SOON HAD TROUBLE SLEEPING...

HIS SPEECHES GREW LISTLESS, HIS FILIBUSTERS LACKLUSTER... UNTIL FINALLY HE SOUGHT PROFESSIONAL HELP.

NOBODY'S OUT TO GET ME!

SINCE THE COLLAPSE OF WORLD COMMUNISM, A DEPRESSED SENATOR HELMS SEEKS PROFESSIONAL HELP WITH HIS ENNUI...

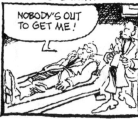

NOBODY'S OUT TO GET ME!

I'VE TRIED BASHING WELFARE CHEATS, LIMO LIBS, FOOD STAMPERS, SECULAR HUMANISTS — IT'S JUST NOT THE SAME ANYMORE!

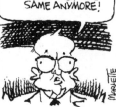

MY RE-ELECTION CAMPAIGN IS SUFFERING!... I'VE EVEN LOST INTEREST IN SMOKING!

SOUNDS LIKE P.M.S!

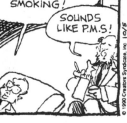

P.M.S.?

POST MACHISMO SYNDROME!

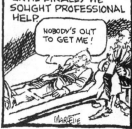

HOLY CATFISH! SENATOR HELMS IS COMING TO BYPASS TO CAMPAIGN!

HE MUST BE DESPERATE!

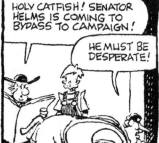

NOBODY COMES TO BYPASS IF THEY DON'T HAVE TO!

POOR JESSE!

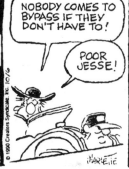

HE'S BEEN LOST SINCE THE COLLAPSE OF COMMUNISM!

MAYBE HE WANTS HIS COLD WAR BUMPER STICKERS SCRAPED!

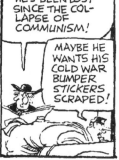

HE SAYS IT'S A SYMBOLIC VISIT!

WE AIN'T GOT NO FLAG FACTORY!

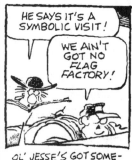

OL' JESSE'S GOT SOMETHING UP HIS SLEEVE!

SENATOR JESSE HELMS SEEKS PROFESSIONAL HELP FOR HIS COLD WAR SEPARATION ANXIETY:

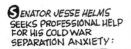

I WANT MY *INTERNATIONAL COMMUNIST CONSPIRACY!*

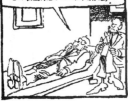

SENATOR, YOU'RE SUFFERING FROM *P.M.S.* — *POST-MACHISMO SYNDROME!* YOU HAVE NO OUTLET FOR YOUR PENT-UP AGGRESSION! I SUGGEST A *HOBBY!*

GOLF... TENNIS... ART...

HMM... ART!

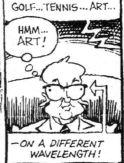

— ON A DIFFERENT WAVELENGTH!

IT'S UP TO ME TO STAND FIRM AGAINST THE EVIL, GODLESS INTERNATIONAL ARTISTIC CONSPIRACY!

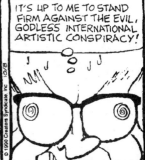

SENATOR JESSE HELMS ON THE RE-ELECTION CAMPAIGN TRAIL WARNS OF THE NEW *POST-COLD WAR MENACE*:

BEWARE THE WICKED *INTERNATIONAL ARTISTIC CONSPIRACY!*

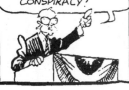

IN THE GOOD OL' DAYS, BACK WHERE I COME FROM, ART WAS SAD-FACED CLOWNS, BIG-EYED CHILDREN AND *BLACK VELVET ELVISES...*

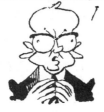

"CULTURE" WAS WHAT THE VETERINARIAN SCRAPED OFF THE COW'S TONGUE TO CHECK FOR HOOF-AND-MOUTH DISEASE...

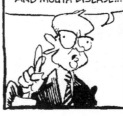

NOW I HAVE NOTHING AGAINST THE SENSITIVE... WHY, SOME OF MY BEST FRIENDS ARE ARTISTS!...

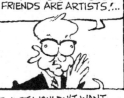

I JUST WOULDN'T WANT ONE MOVING NEXT DOOR OR MARRYING MY DAUGHTER!

SENATOR HELMS CAMPAIGNS AGAINST THE INTERNATIONAL ARTISTIC THREAT.

THEY'LL TURN OUR CHILDREN INTO TURPENTINE ADDICTS AND *LINSEED OIL JUNKIES!*

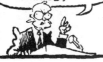

FEDERAL GRANTS WILL LEAD TO ABSTRACT EXPRESSIONISM, THESPIANISM, AND *ALTERNATIVE LIFESTYLES!*

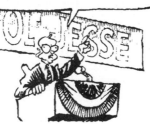

RE-ELECT JESSE HELMS!... AND REMEMBER: A MIND IS A *TERRIBLE THING...*

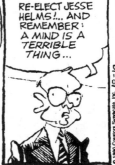

... PERIOD.

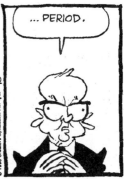

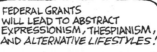

SENATOR HELMS' GUIDE TO THE INTERNATIONAL ARTISTIC CONSPIRACY...

THEY KNOW WHO THEY ARE!

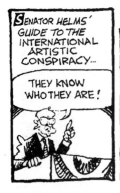

HOW TO RECOGNIZE ARTISTS, THESPIANS, AND FELLOW-TRAVELERS:

THEY OFTEN DRESS IN BLACK LEOTARDS, ...AND SMELL OF LINSEED OIL!...

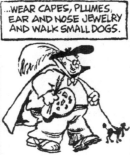

...WEAR CAPES, PLUMES, EAR AND NOSE JEWELRY AND WALK SMALL DOGS.

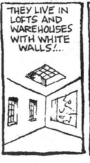

THEY LIVE IN LOFTS AND WAREHOUSES WITH WHITE WALLS!...

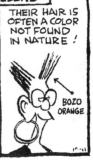

THEIR HAIR IS OFTEN A COLOR NOT FOUND IN NATURE!

BOZO ORANGE

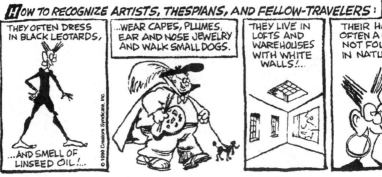

SENATOR HELMS' INTERNATIONAL ARTISTIC CONSPIRACY BLACKLIST! THE TELLTALE TRAITS OF ARTISTS, THESPIANS AND OTHER SO-CALLED "CREATIVE-TYPES."

YOU KNOW WHO YOU ARE!

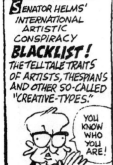

ULTRA-SENSITIVE...

WHAT A SNIFF LOVELY SUNSET!... I THINK I SHALL WEEP!

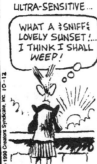

PALE, WAN, "SICKLY"...

HONK

YEATS

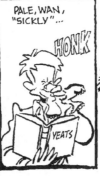

WRITES 'THANK-YOU' NOTES...

...IN CALLIGRAPHY!

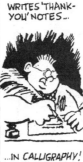

...BLUDGEONS OTHERS WITH HIS/HER EXQUISITE TASTE...

LOSE THE VASE!

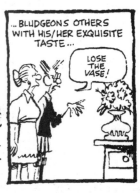

JESSE HELMS DEBATES HIS SENATORIAL OPPONENT...

ARE YOU NOW, OR HAVE YOU EVER BEEN A MEMBER OF THE BOOK-OF-THE-MONTH CLUB?

HOLY CATFISH! OL' JESSE'S SURE MILKING THIS ANTI-CULTURE THING!

BETTER DEAD THAN WELL-READ!

NO SKIN OFF MY BACK!

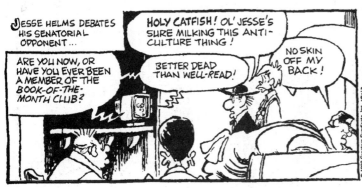

FAMOUS LAST WORDS...

WELCOME TO BYPASS BLACK VELVET ART CAPITOL OF THE WORLD

JESSE

US SENATE

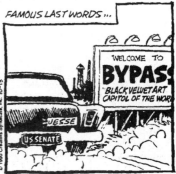

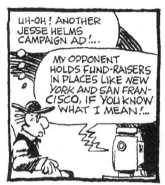

UH-OH! ANOTHER JESSE HELMS CAMPAIGN AD!...

MY OPPONENT HOLDS FUND-RAISERS IN PLACES LIKE NEW YORK AND SAN FRANCISCO, IF YOU KNOW WHAT I MEAN!...

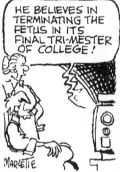

HE BELIEVES IN TERMINATING THE FETUS IN ITS FINAL TRI-MESTER OF COLLEGE!

MARLETTE

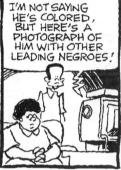

I'M NOT SAYING HE'S COLORED, BUT HERE'S A PHOTOGRAPH OF HIM WITH OTHER LEADING NEGROES!

© 1990 Creators Syndicate, Inc. 10/15

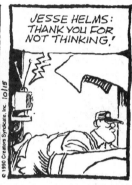

JESSE HELMS: THANK YOU FOR NOT THINKING!

BYPASS, THE "FLORENCE" OF MOZELLE COUNTY, HAS ALWAYS SUPPORTED THE ARTS...

FROM STREET BLUES...

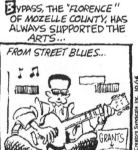

GRANTS

© 1990 Creators Syndicate, Inc. 10/16

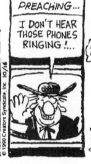

..TO TV PREACHING...

I DON'T HEAR THOSE PHONES RINGING!...

KEROSENE

MARLETTE

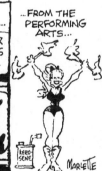

...FROM THE PERFORMING ARTS...

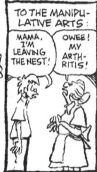

TO THE MANIPULATIVE ARTS:

MAMA, I'M LEAVING THE NEST!

OWEE! MY ARTHRITIS!

...ITS "CREATIVE-TYPES" ARE ENCOURAGED TO FORGE IN THE SMITHY OF THEIR SOULS THE UNCREATED CONSCIENCE OF THE RACE...

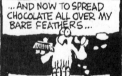

...AND NOW TO SPREAD CHOCOLATE ALL OVER MY BARE FEATHERS...

...TO PROTEST DISCRIMINATION AGAINST PARAKEETS!

SENATOR JESSE HELMS' BLACK VELVET ART COLLECTION:

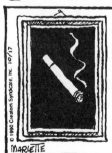

© 1990 Creators Syndicate, Inc. 10/17

MARLETTE

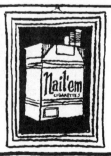

Nail'em CIGARETTES

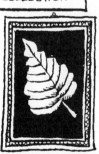

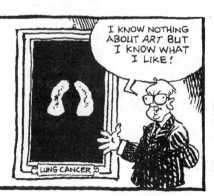

LUNG CANCER

I KNOW NOTHING ABOUT ART BUT I KNOW WHAT I LIKE!

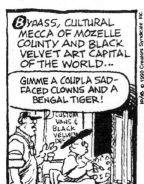

BYPASS, CULTURAL MECCA OF MOZELLE COUNTY AND BLACK VELVET ART CAPITAL OF THE WORLD...

GIMME A COUPLA SAD-FACED CLOWNS AND A BENGAL TIGER!

CUSTOM VANS & BLACK VELVET

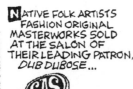

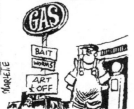

NATIVE FOLK ARTISTS FASHION ORIGINAL MASTERWORKS SOLD AT THE SALON OF THEIR LEADING PATRON, DUB DUBOSE...

GAS

BAIT WORMS

ART ¢ OFF

© 1990 Creators Syndicate, Inc.

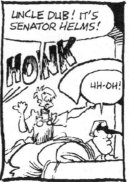

UNCLE DUB! IT'S SENATOR HELMS!

HONK

UH-OH!

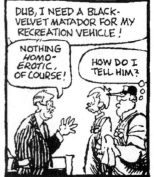

DUB, I NEED A BLACK-VELVET MATADOR FOR MY RECREATION VEHICLE!

NOTHING HOMO-EROTIC, OF COURSE!

HOW DO I TELL HIM?

BYPASS, THE "PARIS" OF BLACK VELVET ART...

DUB DUBOSE, GALLERY OWNER

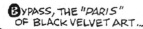

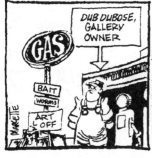

GAS

BAIT WORMS

ART OFF

© 1990 Creators Syndicate, Inc. 10/19

ANONYMOUS CLASSICS SOLD HERE ADORN THE WALLS OF CHEAP MOTELS, APARTMENT COMPLEXES, DENTIST OFFICES...

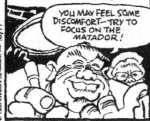

YOU MAY FEEL SOME DISCOMFORT—TRY TO FOCUS ON THE MATADOR!

...AND UNTIL NOW, SENATORIAL RECREATION VEHICLES...

WHAT DO YOU MEAN YOU'RE ALL OUT!?

ZIP!

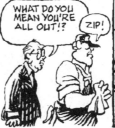

I SMELL THE INTERNATIONAL ARTISTIC CON-SPIRACY! THIS CALLS FOR A WITCH-HU—ER—HEARING!

RIGHT HERE IN BYPASS?!

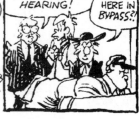

ON A SYMBOLIC CAMPAIGN STOP IN BLACK VELVET ART MECCA, BYPASS, SENATOR HELMS IS STUNNED TO HEAR:

SORRY—WE'RE ALL OUT!

OUT!?

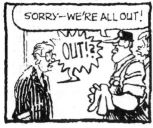

THE NATIONAL ENDOWMENT FOR THE ARTS SUBSIDIZES US NOW NOT TO PRODUCE BLACK VELVET ARTWORK!

© 1990 Creators Syndicate, Inc. 10/20

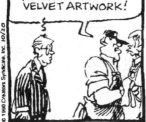

ALL THE BLACK VELVET PAINTINGS IN BYPASS ARE ROTTING IN SILOS!...

EXCEPT FOR MY ELVIS!

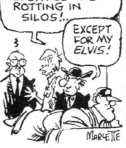

WH-WHY, THAT'S CENSORSHIP!

—OR GOOD TASTE!

..OR BOTH!

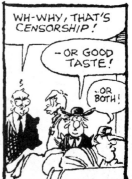

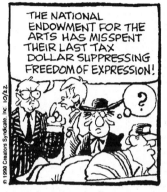

WHAT?! THE NATIONAL ENDOWMENT FOR THE ARTS SUBSIDIZES BYPASS ARTISTS *NOT* TO CREATE BLACK VELVET ARTWORK!

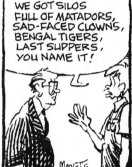

WE GOT SILOS FULL OF MATADORS, SAD-FACED CLOWNS, BENGAL TIGERS, LAST SUPPERS, YOU NAME IT!

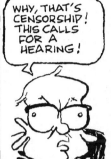

WHY, THAT'S CENSORSHIP! THIS CALLS FOR A HEARING!

© 1990 Creators Syndicate, Inc 10/22

THE NATIONAL ENDOWMENT FOR THE ARTS HAS MISSPENT THEIR LAST TAX DOLLAR SUPPRESSING FREEDOM OF EXPRESSION!

?

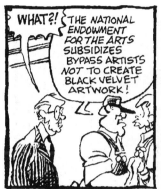

HELMS INVESTIGATES ARTS FUNDING IN BYPASS:

I DO EAR WAX SCULPTURE AND I COULDN'T GET A GRANT.

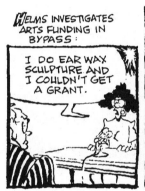

I AM A DRIVER'S LICENSE PHOTOGRAPHER, AND THE NATIONAL ENDOWMENT REFUSED TO FUND AN EXHIBIT OF MY WORK.

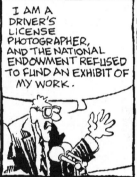

I AM A COSMETIC SURGEON INTO FACIAL ABSTRACT EXPRESSIONISM, AND I WAS TURNED DOWN.

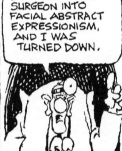

I AM A BLACK VELVET ARTIST, AND THE *NEA* PAID ME *NOT* TO SHOW MY WORK!

OUTRAGEOUS!

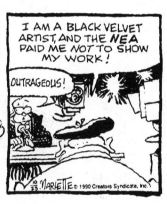

10/23 MARLETTE © 1990 Creators Syndicate, Inc

SENATOR HELMS HOLDS A HEARING IN BYPASS:

NAME:

NASAL T. LARDBOTTOM.

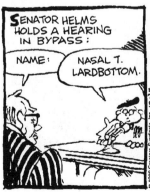

OCCUPATION:

BLACK VELVET ARTISTE.

© 1990 Creators Syndicate, Inc 10-24

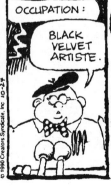

...AND WHERE IS YOUR WORK EXHIBITED?

NOWHERE. NOW.

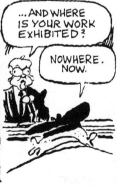

THE NATIONAL ENDOWMENT FOR THE ARTS SUBSIDIZES ME TO STORE IT IN A SILO ON THE OUTSKIRTS OF TOWN!

WELL, I SAY IT'S TIME FOR A SHOW!

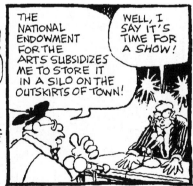

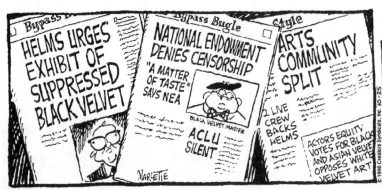

HELMS URGES EXHIBIT OF SUPPRESSED BLACK VELVET

Bypass Bugle

NATIONAL ENDOWMENT DENIES CENSORSHIP

"A MATTER OF TASTE" SAYS NEA

BLACK VELVET MASTER

ACLU SILENT

Style

ARTS COMMUNITY SPLIT

2 LIVE CREW BACKS HELMS

ACTORS EQUITY VOTES FOR BLACK AND ASIAN VELVET OPPOSES WHITE VELVET ART

ON THE EVE OF THE SHOW HELMS IS GLOATING:

ARE YOU SURE YOU DON'T WANT TO SEE THE EXHIBIT BEFOREHAND, SENATOR?

WHY?! YOU SEEN ONE PAINTING YOU SEEN 'EM ALL!

© 1990 Creators Syndicate, Inc. 10-25

A SHOW OF SUPPRESSED BLACK VELVET ART IS UNVEILED BY CONNOISSEUR *JESSE HELMS.*

VOILA!

© 1990 Creators Syndicate, Inc. 10-24

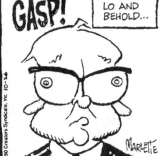

GASP!

LO AND BEHOLD...

A PHOTO OF SENATOR HELMS SUBMERGED IN TOBACCO JUICE ENTITLED *"SPIT HELMS"*!

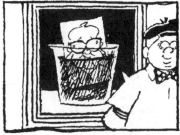

SENATOR JESSE HELMS FINDS HIMSELF IN THE AWKWARD POSITION OF DEFENDING THE BLACK VELVET MASTERPIECE *"SPIT HELMS"*!...

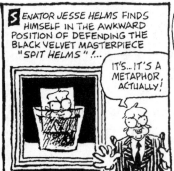

IT'S...IT'S A METAPHOR, ACTUALLY!

...ER...A SYMBOLIC EXPRESSION... UH... OF THE HUMAN PREDICAMENT...

IT'S NOT MEANT TO BE TAKEN LITERALLY!

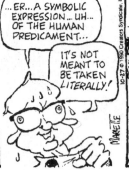

OL' JESSE'S SQUIRMIN'...

FOR THE FIRST TIME IN HIS LIFE HE CAN'T BLAME COMMIES, LIBERALS, WELFARE CHEATS, GAYS, BLACKS, ARTISTS...

HE CAN'T BLAME NOBODY BUT HIS OWN SELF!

AMEN!

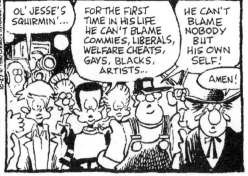

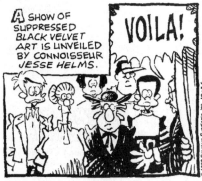

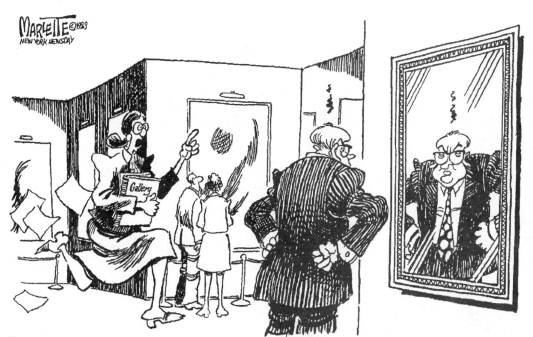

"NO, SENATOR HELMS, THAT'S NOT A *MAPPLETHORPE* — THAT'S A *MIRROR!*"

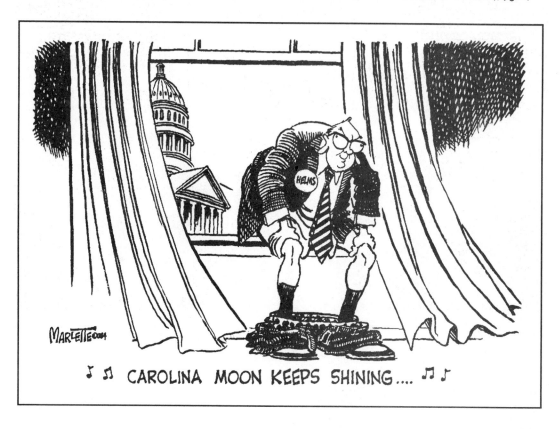

♪ ♫ CAROLINA MOON KEEPS SHINING.... ♫ ♪

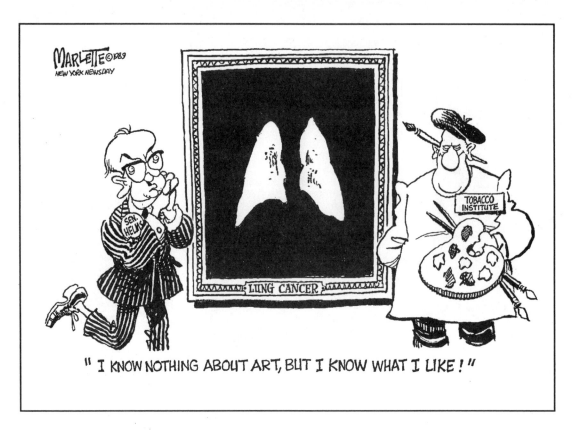

" I KNOW NOTHING ABOUT ART, BUT I KNOW WHAT I LIKE ! "

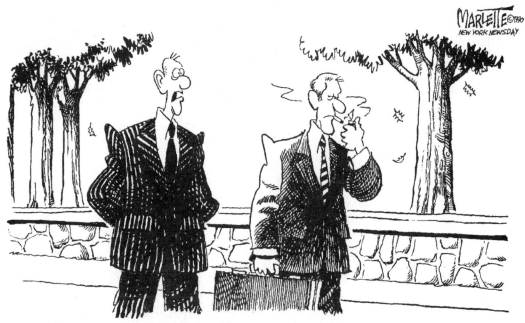

"LUNG CANCER ?... NO, I QUIT WHEN I LEARNED TOBACCO'S LINKED TO *JESSE HELMS!*"

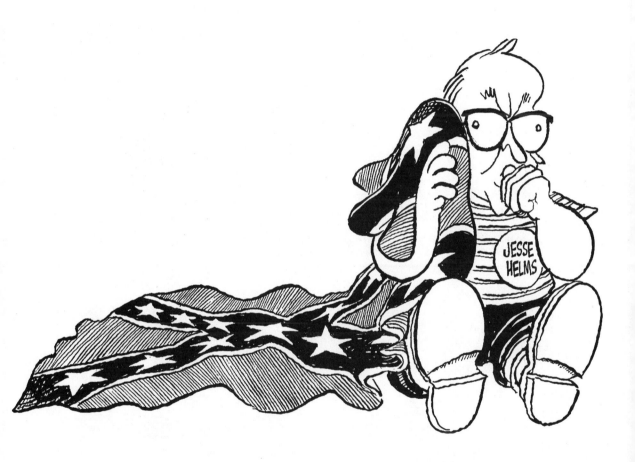

LOOSE LIPS SINK CHAIRMANSHIPS!

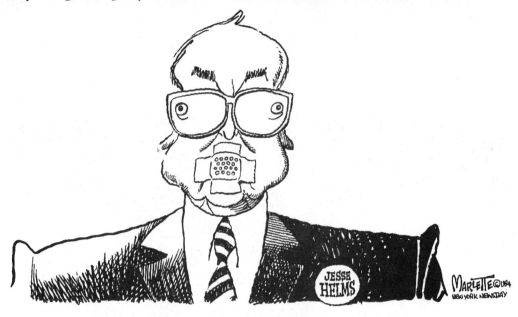

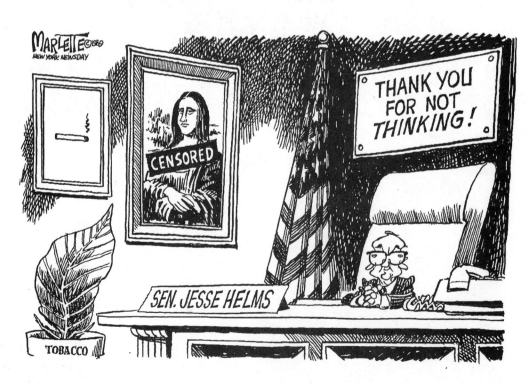

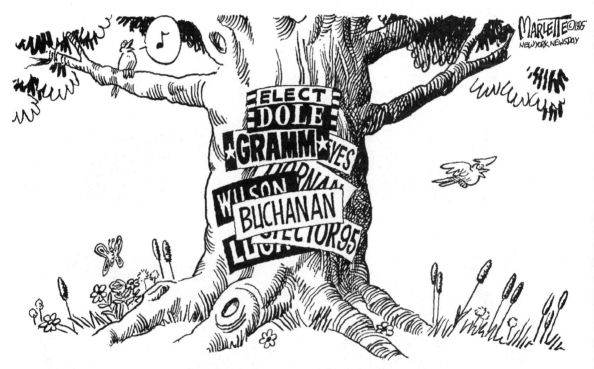

ELECT
DOLE
GRAMM ★YES
WILSON
BUCHANAN
LUGLECTOR 95

Springtime: When The Saps Rise...

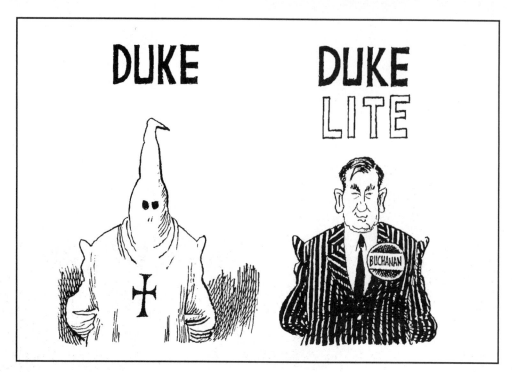

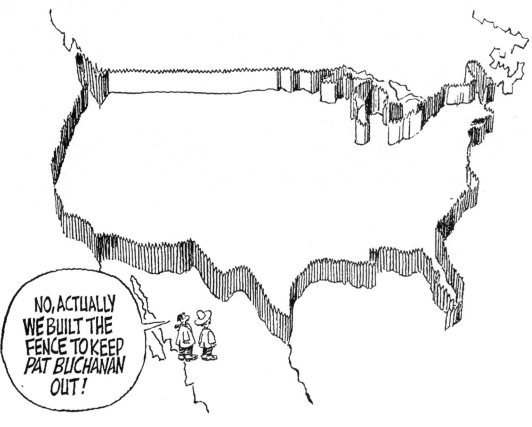

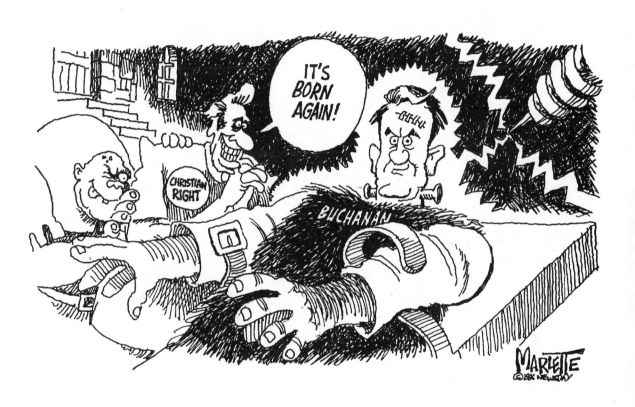

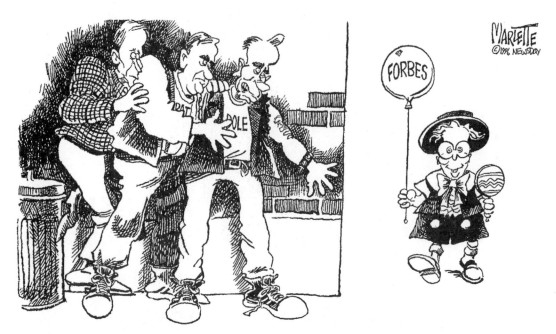

"HERE COMES THAT BIG BULLY NOW!"

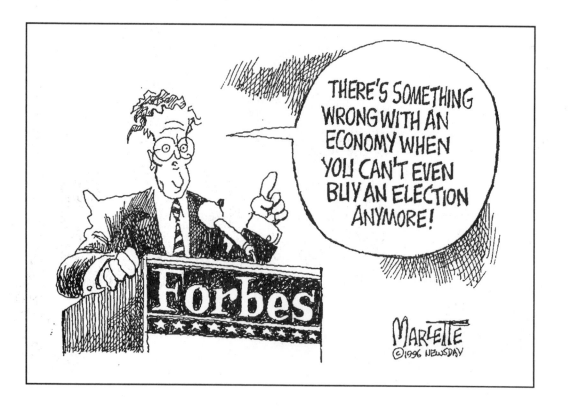

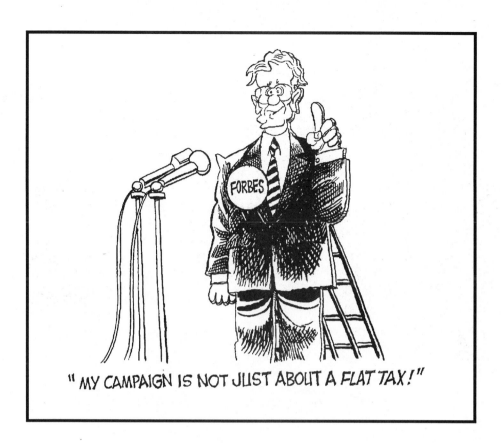

" MY CAMPAIGN IS NOT JUST ABOUT A *FLAT TAX!* "

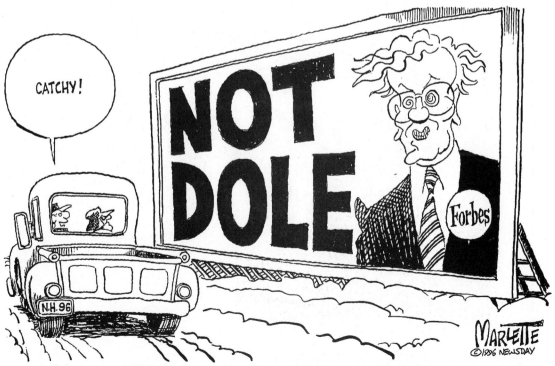

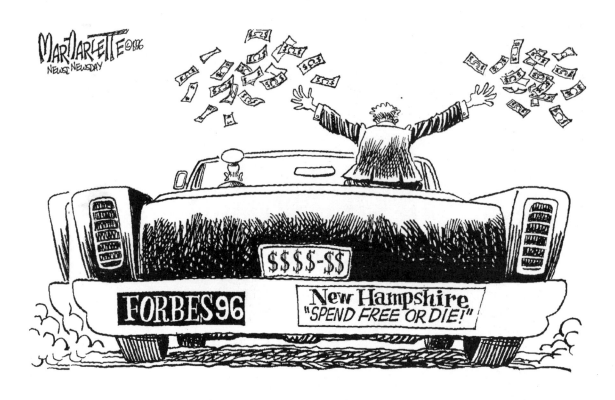

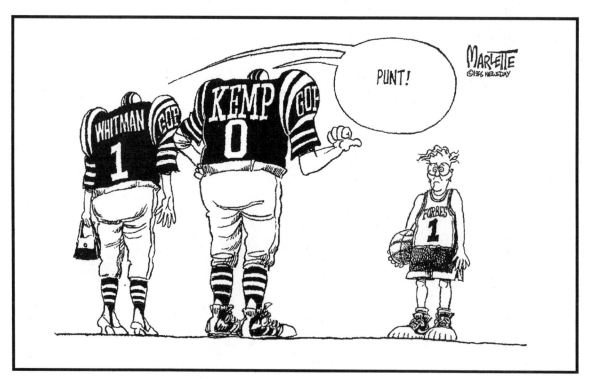

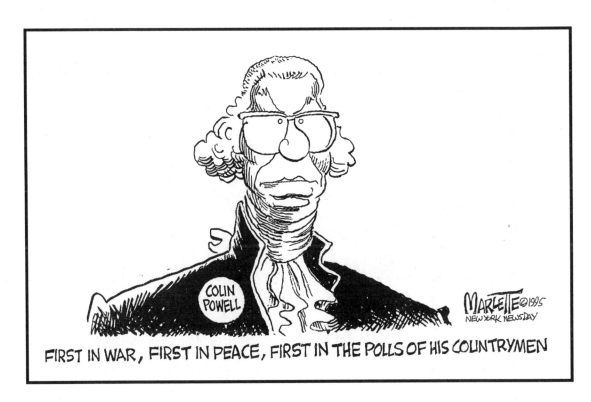

FIRST IN WAR, FIRST IN PEACE, FIRST IN THE POLLS OF HIS COUNTRYMEN

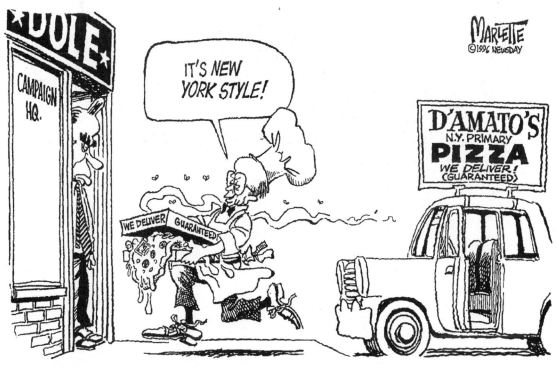

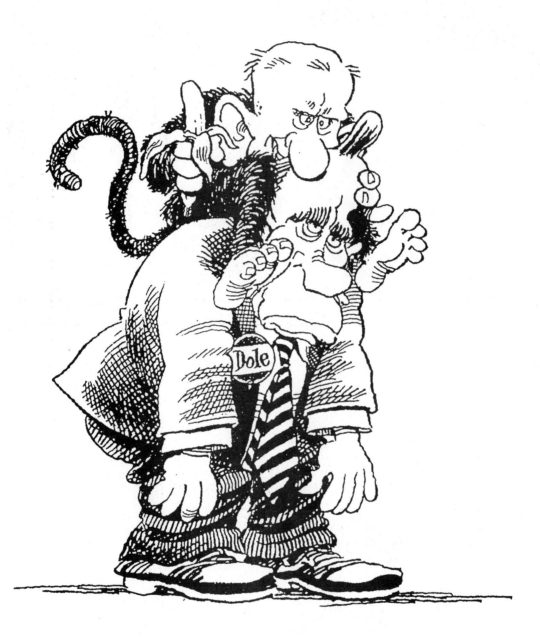

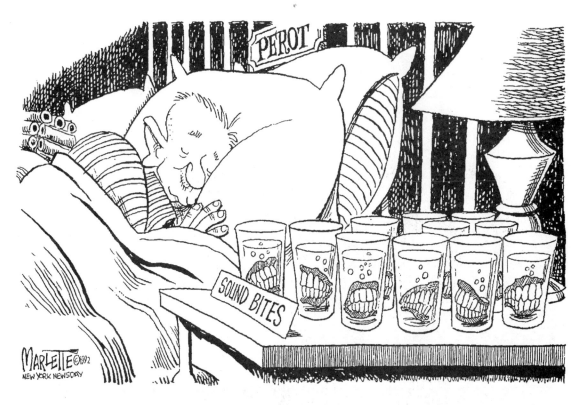

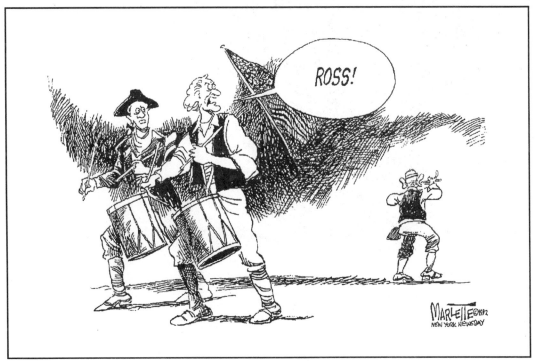

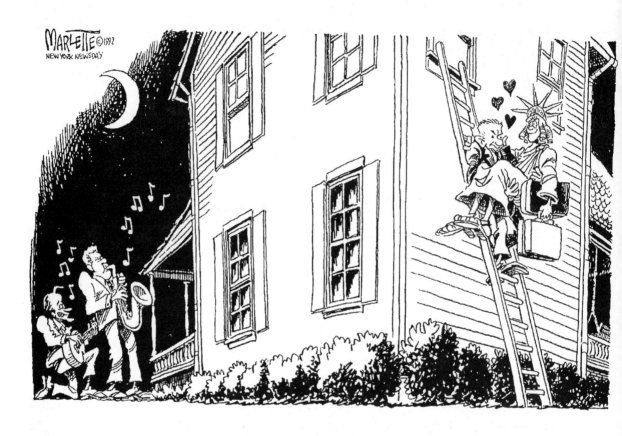

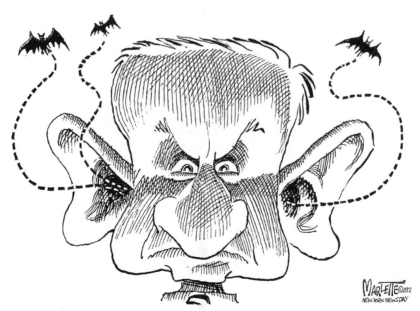

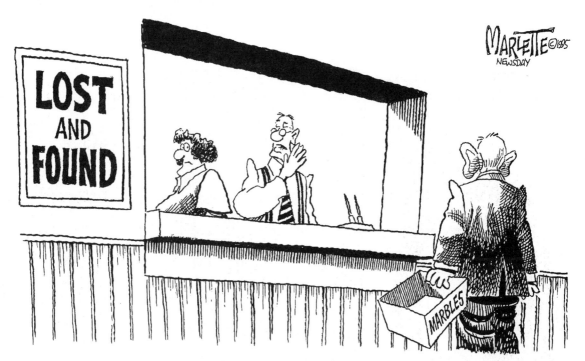

"IT'S ROSS PEROT AGAIN!"

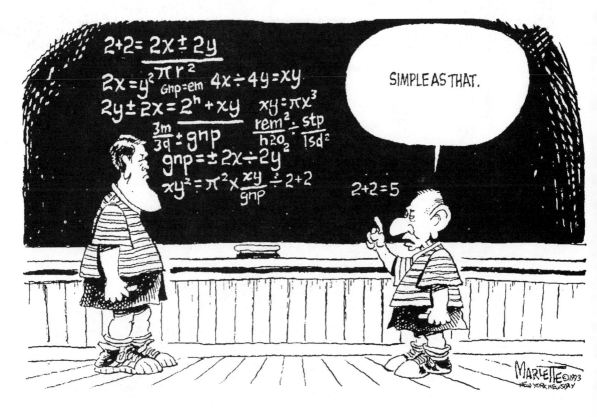

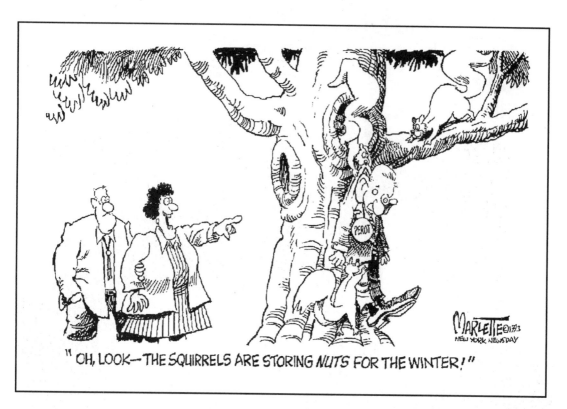

"OH, LOOK—THE SQUIRRELS ARE STORING *NUTS* FOR THE WINTER!"

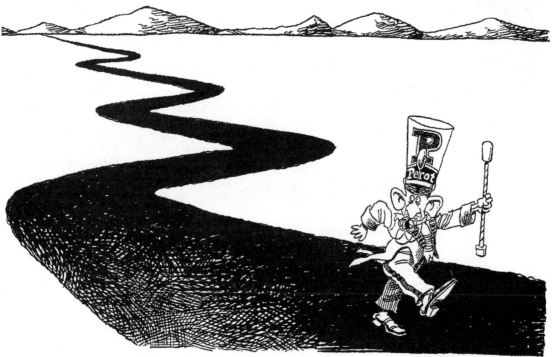

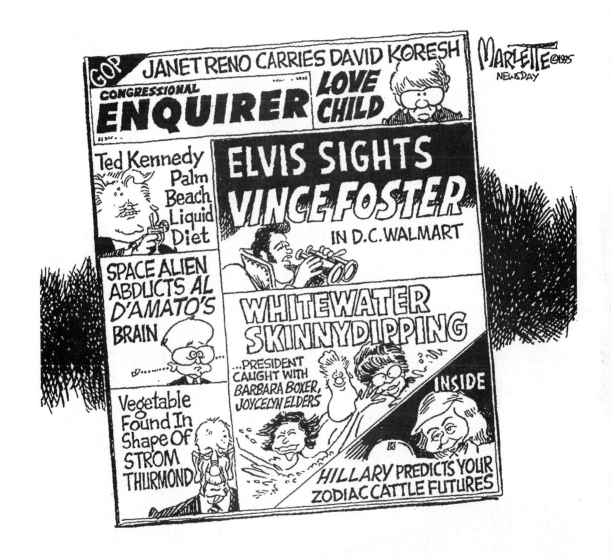

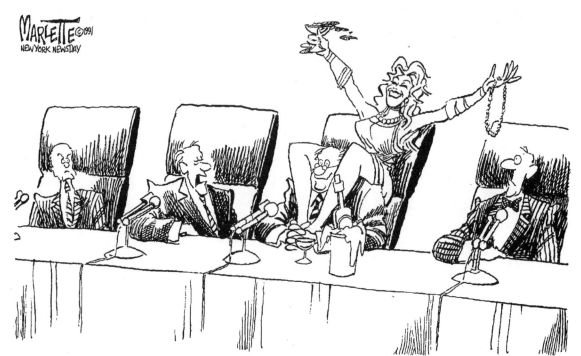

"A SYSTEM OF *CHECKS* AND BALANCES, SENATOR — NOT *CHICKS* AND BALANCES!..."

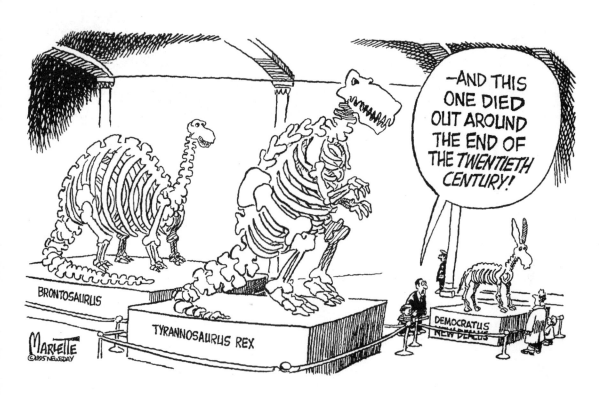

RESULT OF BURNING THE *ETERNAL FLAME* AT BOTH ENDS:

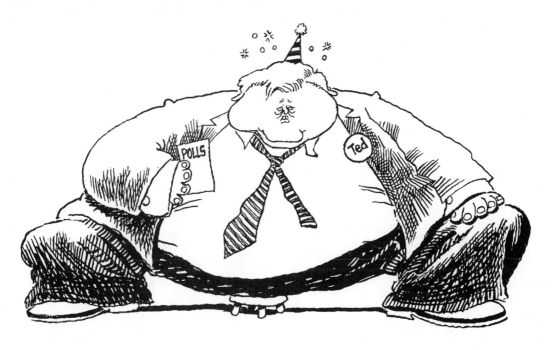

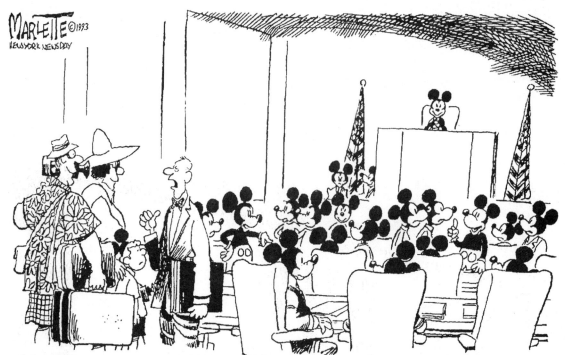

"THE NEW DISNEY THEME PARK?...NO, THIS IS JUST THE *U.S. CONGRESS!*"

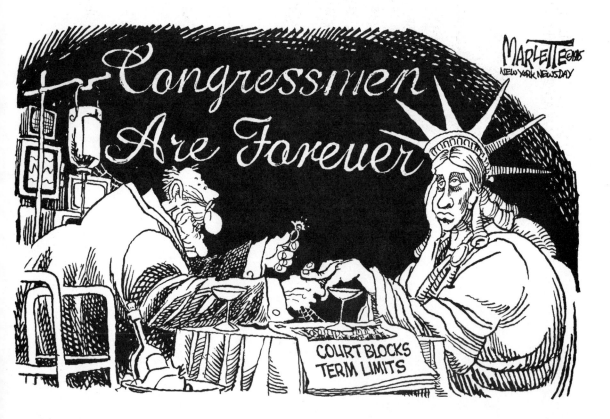

Congressmen Are Forever

COURT BLOCKS TERM LIMITS

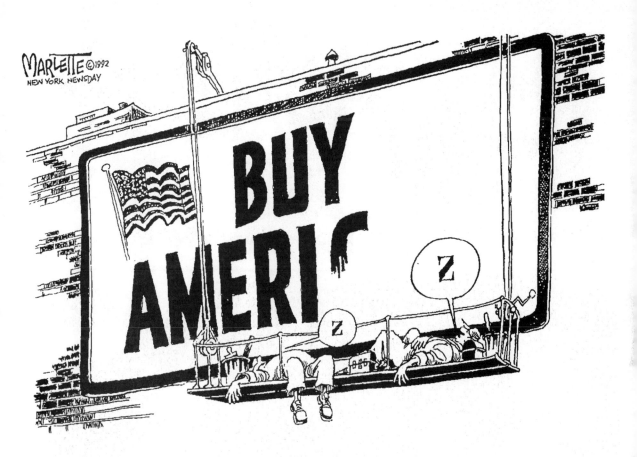

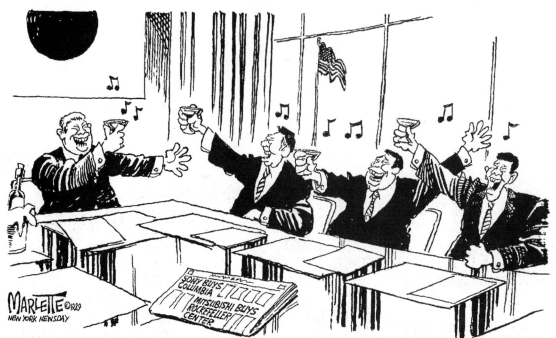

"...THIS LAND IS YOUR LAND!...THIS LAND IS MY LAND!... FROM CALIFORNIA... TO THE NEW YORK ISLANDS!..."

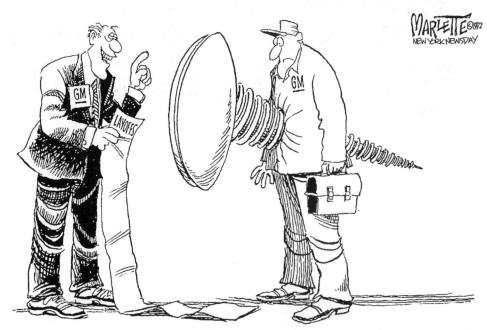

" YOU'LL BE PLEASED TO KNOW THAT *PART* WAS MADE IN THE *U.S.A..!*"

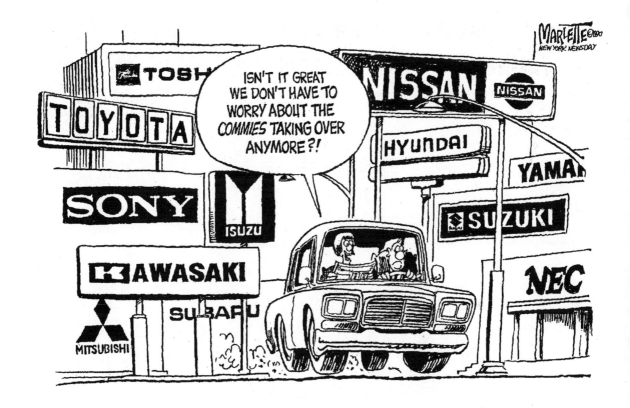

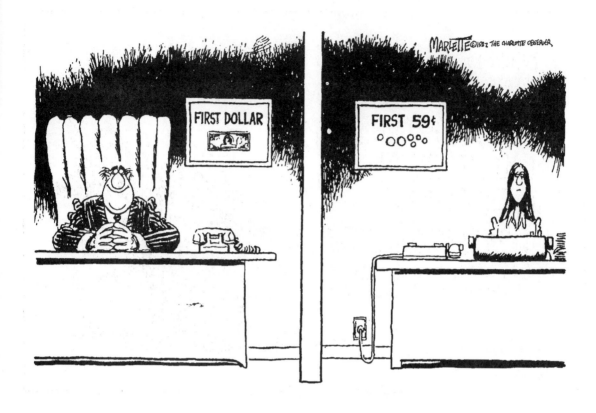

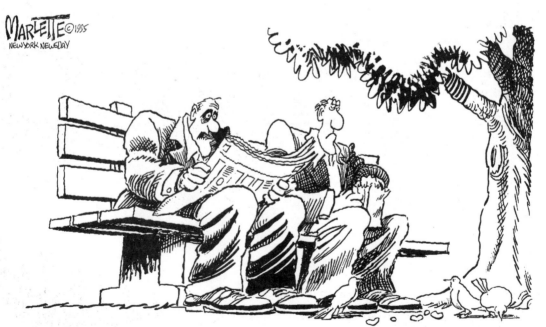

"...SO I TOOK MY DAUGHTER TO WORK, THEY HIRED HER AT HALF MY SALARY AND FIRED ME!"

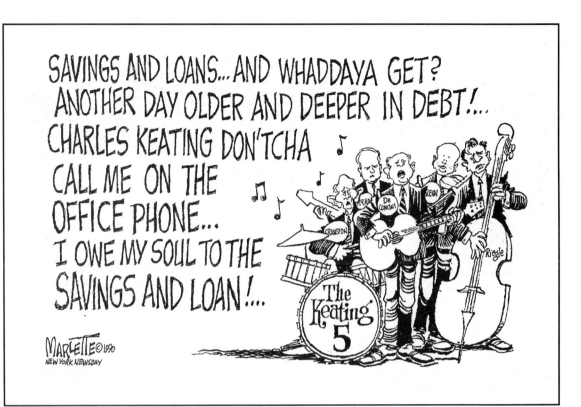

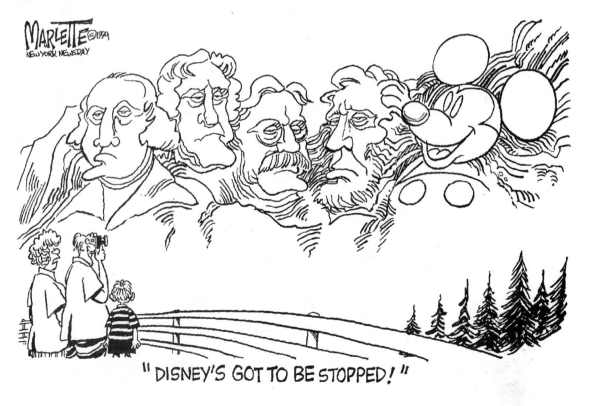

"DISNEY'S GOT TO BE STOPPED!"

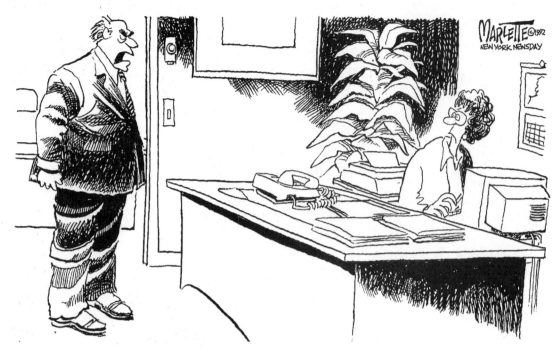

"YOU FORGOT TO REMIND ME IT'S *NATIONAL SECRETARY'S WEEK* — YOU'RE *FIRED!*"

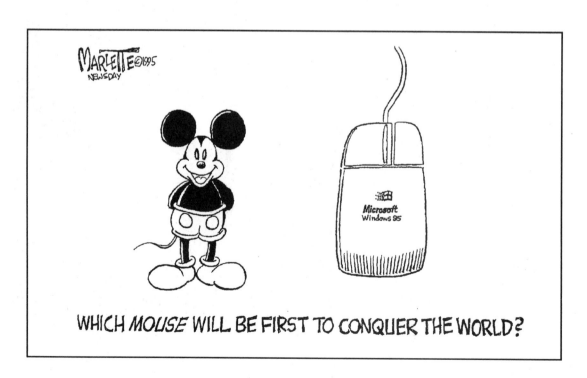

WHICH *MOUSE* WILL BE FIRST TO CONQUER THE WORLD?

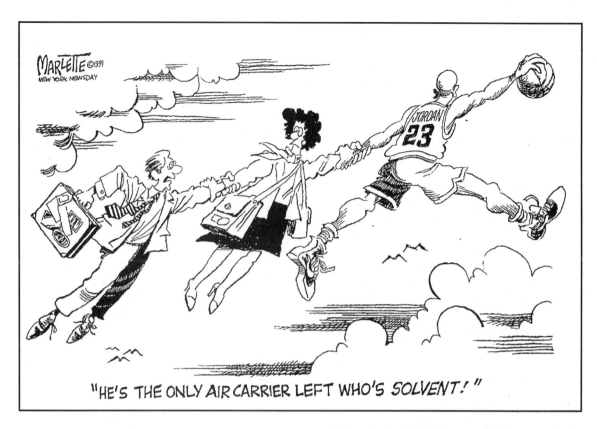

"HE'S THE ONLY AIR CARRIER LEFT WHO'S *SOLVENT!*"

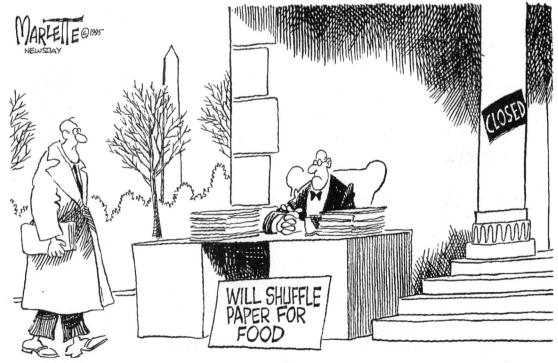

WILL SHUFFLE
PAPER FOR
FOOD

CLOSED

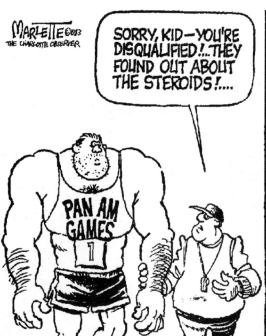

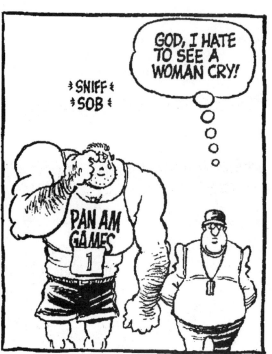

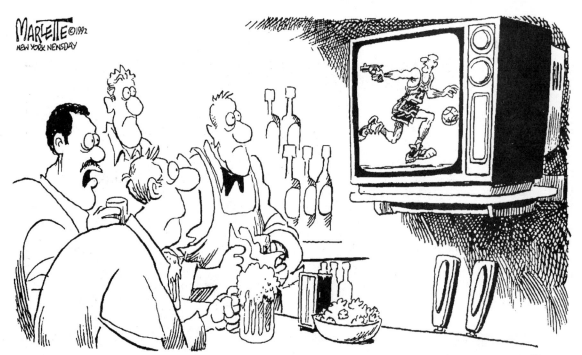

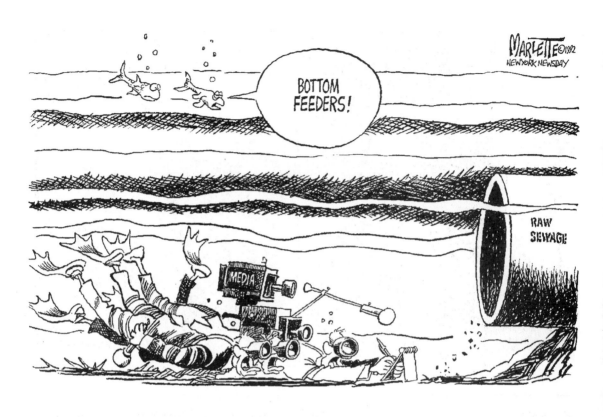

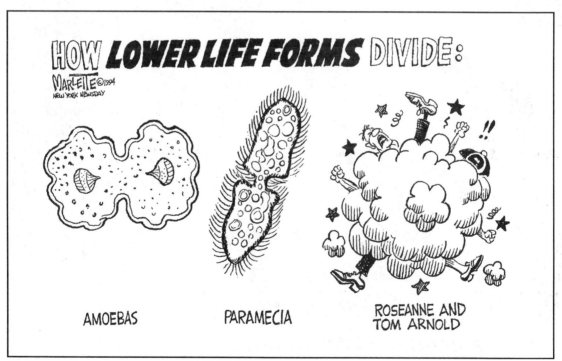

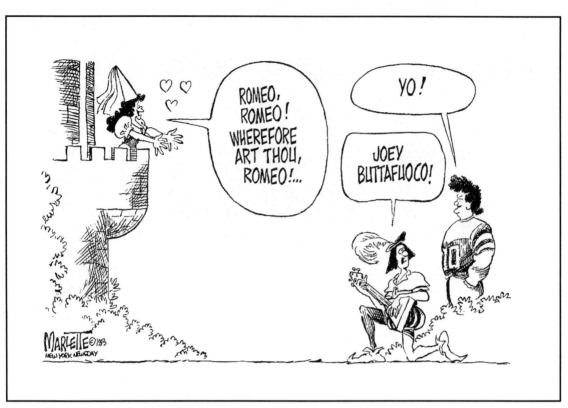

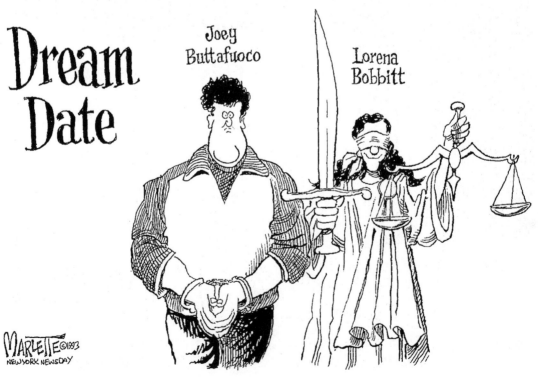

Dream Date

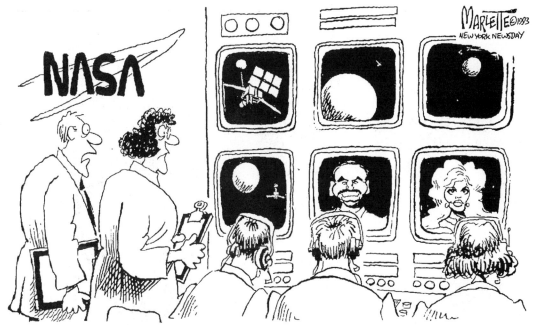

"WE LOST CONTACT WITH THE MARS PROBE, BUT WE STILL CAN'T SHAKE *BURT* AND *LONI!*"

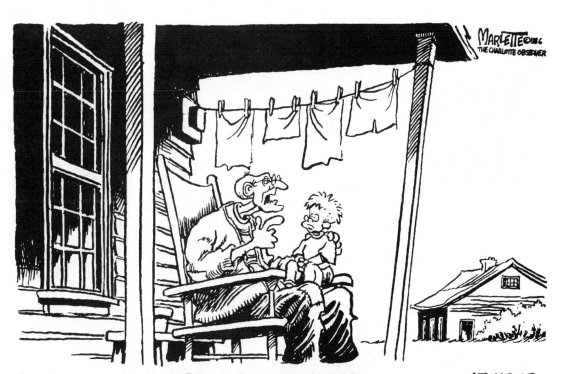

"WHY, WHEN I WAS A BOY WE WERE SO BAD OFF WE DIDN'T HAVE A SINGLE CELEBRITY INTERESTED IN OUR PLIGHT!"

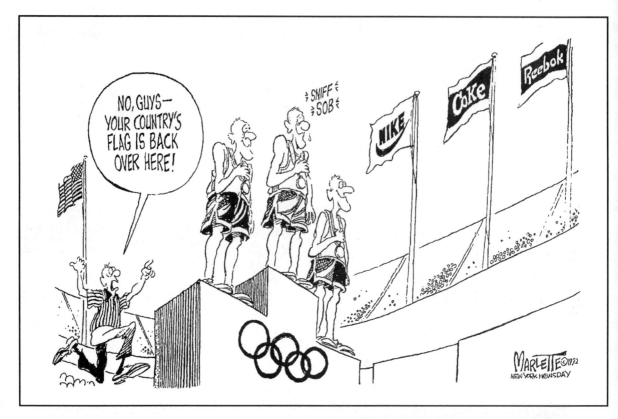

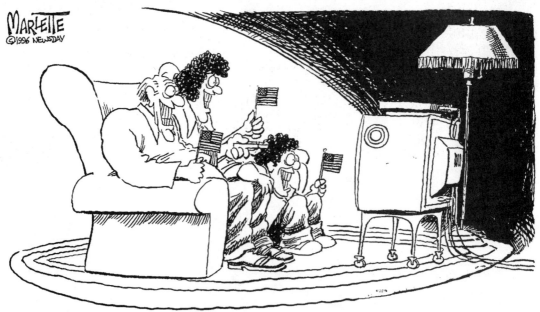

"...AND THE AMERICANS GO FOR THE GOLD IN THE *ATTENTION SPAN VAULT* WITH A RECORD-BREAKING HOP, SKIP AND JUMP FROM THE *VALUJET* CRASH TO THE *TWA FLIGHT 800* EXPLOSION TO THE *CENTENNIAL PARK BOMBING!*..."

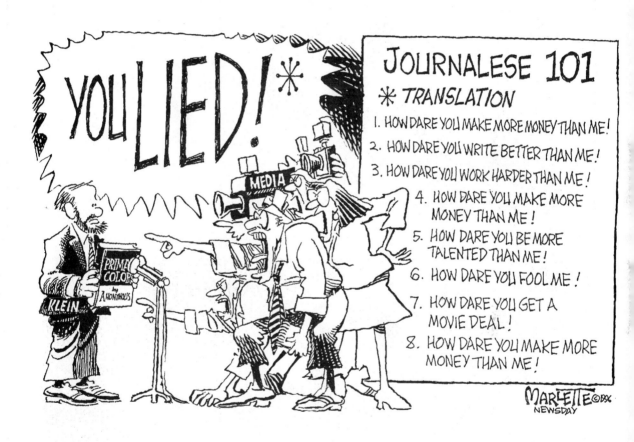

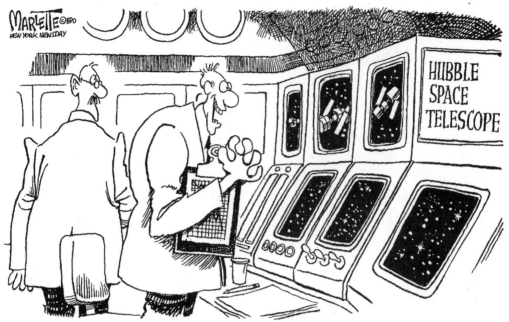

"EUREKA! I CAN SEE THE END OF THE *NBA PLAYOFFS!*"

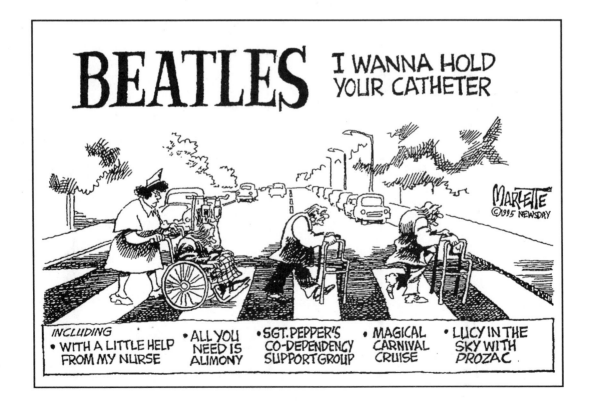

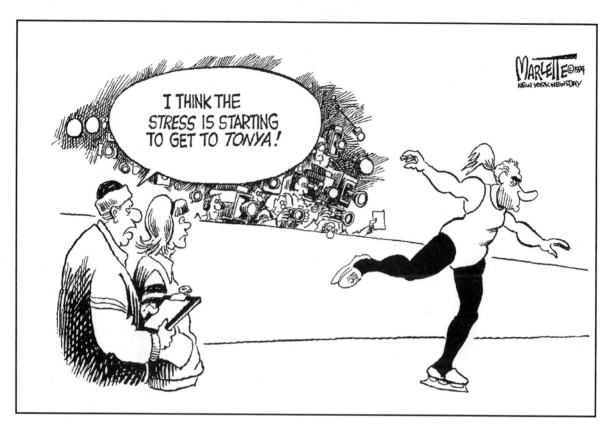

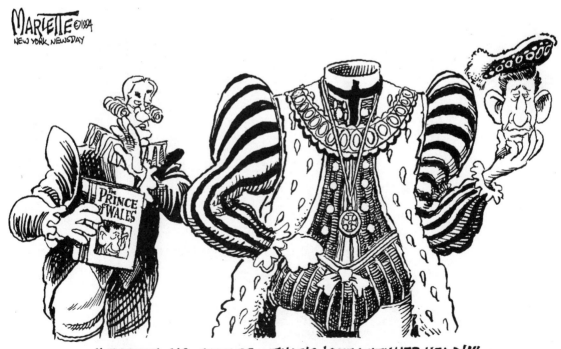

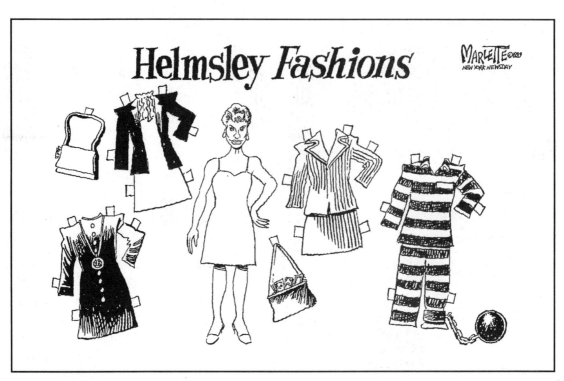

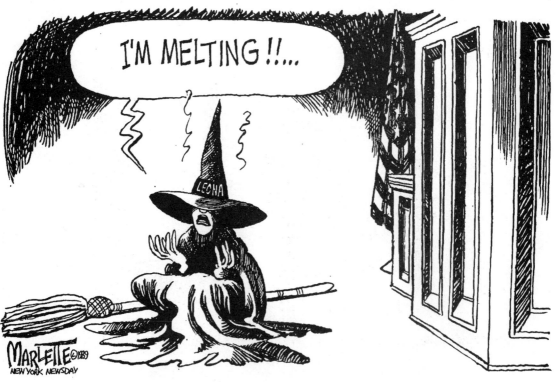

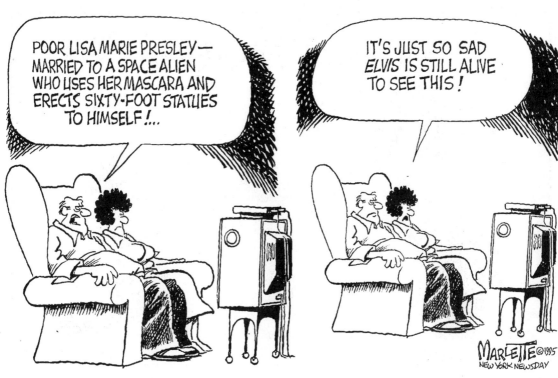

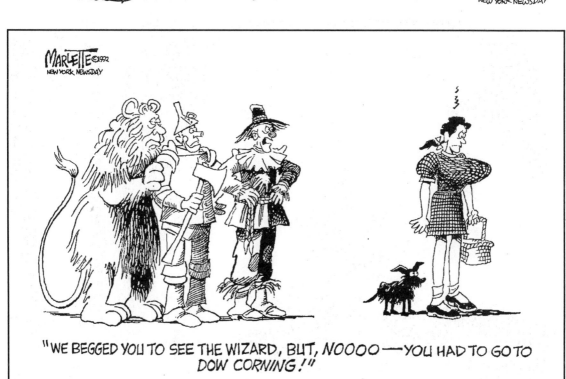

"WE BEGGED YOU TO SEE THE WIZARD, BUT, NOOOO —YOU HAD TO GO TO DOW CORNING!"

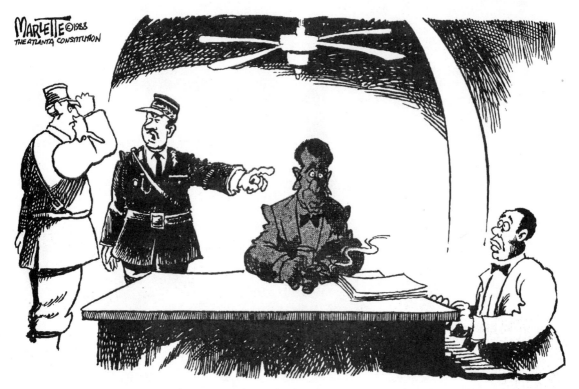

"BOGEY'S BEEN *COLORIZED!* ROUND UP THE USUAL SUSPECTS!"

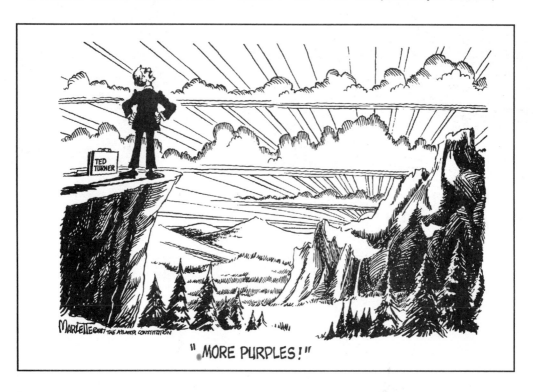

".MORE PURPLES!"

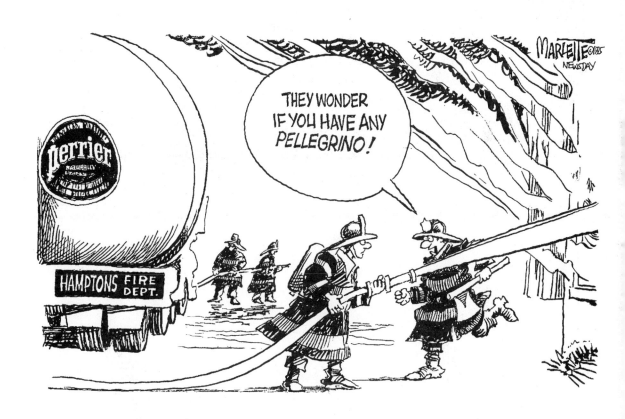

127

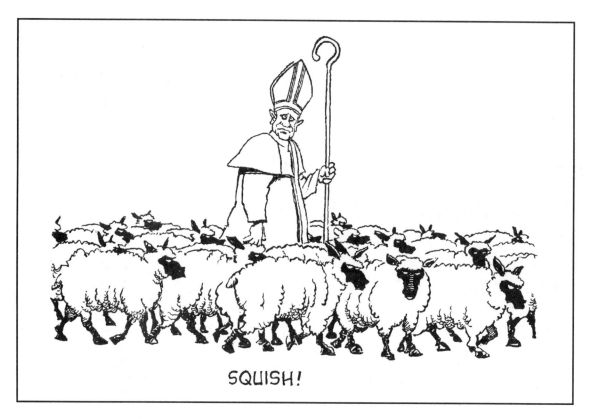

SQUISH!

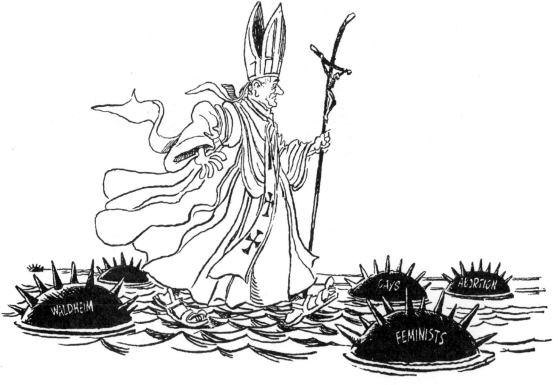

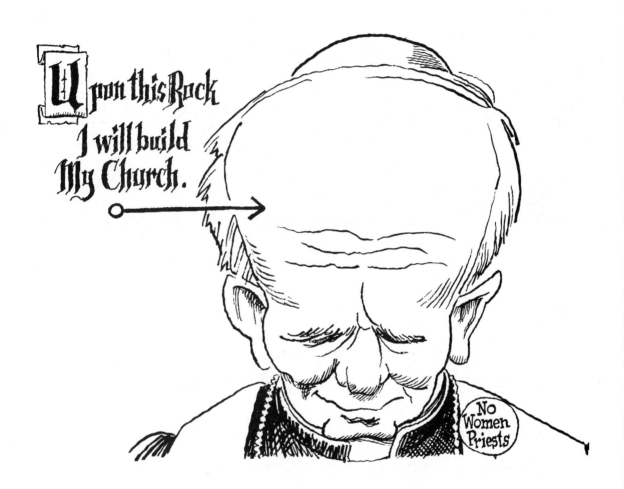

Upon this Rock I will build My Church.

No Women Priests

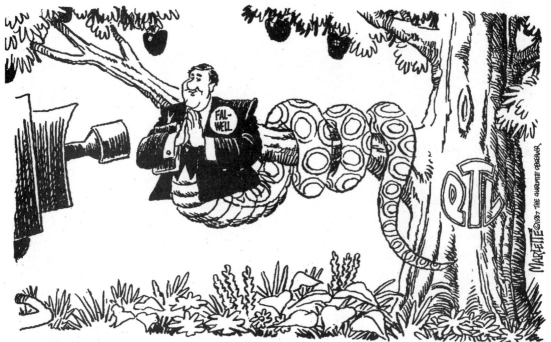

"THAT'S RIGHT — JIM AND TAMMY WERE EXPELLED FROM PARADISE AND LEFT ME IN CHARGE!"

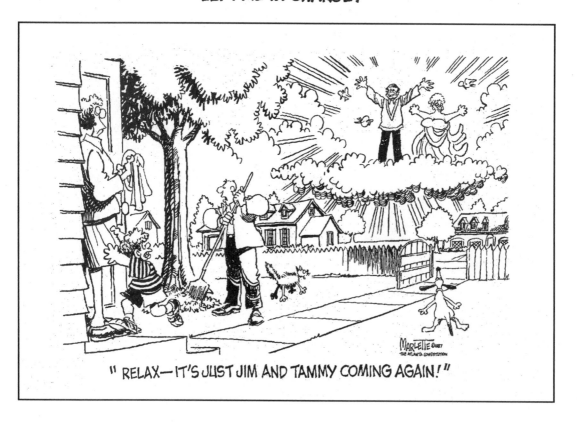

"RELAX — IT'S JUST JIM AND TAMMY COMING AGAIN!"

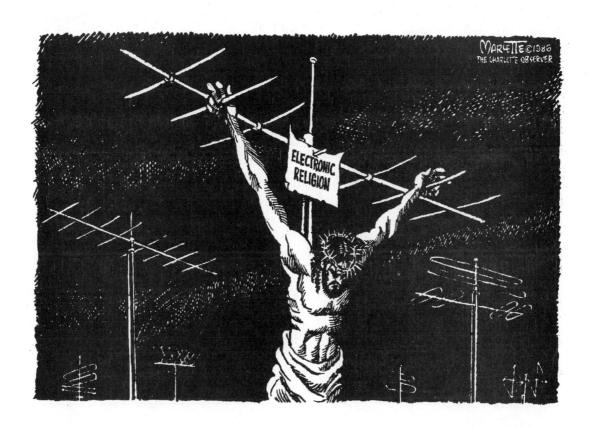

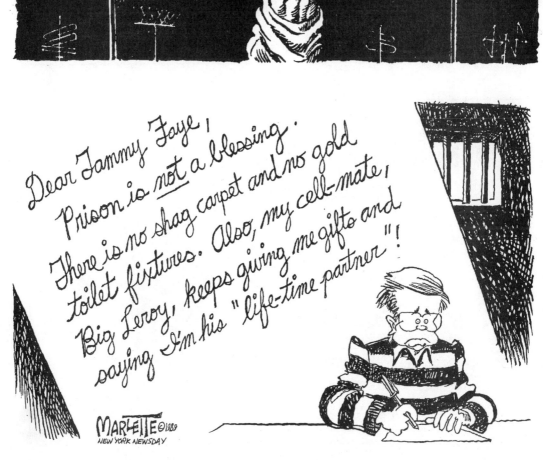

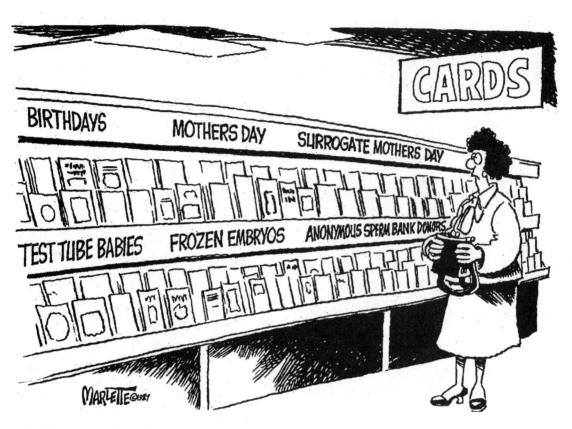

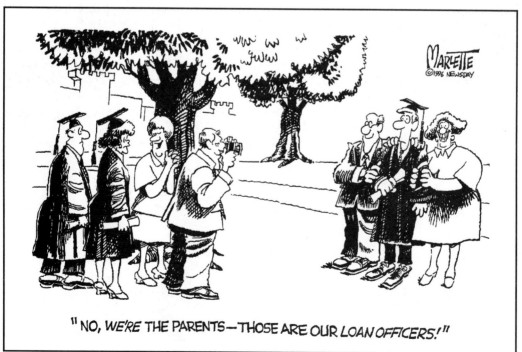

"NO, WE'RE THE PARENTS—THOSE ARE OUR *LOAN OFFICERS!*"

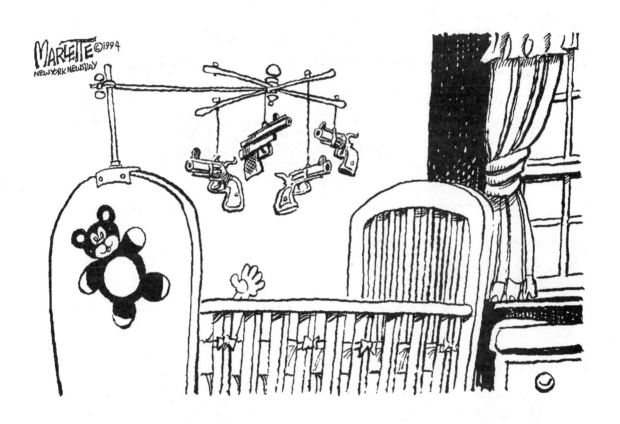

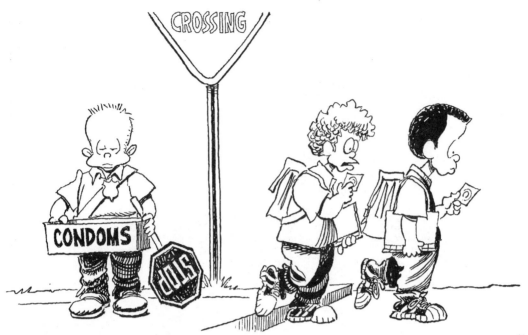

"REMEMBER WHEN THE *SAFETY PATROL* JUST HELPED US CROSS THE STREET !..."

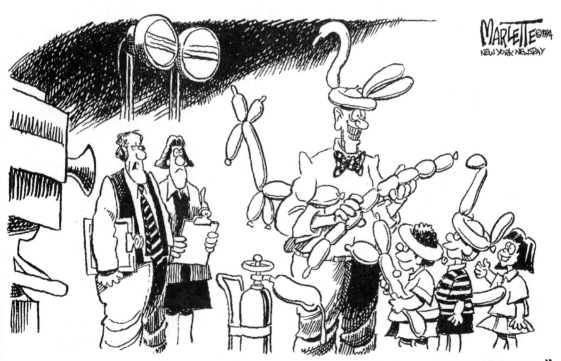

"FRANKLY, I THINK WE'VE CROSSED THE LINE WITH THESE CONDOM ADS FOR KIDS !..."

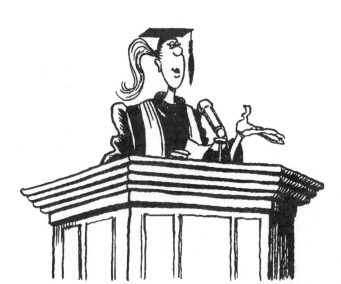

"AS, LIKE, CLASS VALEDICTORIAN, YOU KNOW, I WAS TRYING TO THINK, YOU KNOW, IN MY HEAD, LIKE, WHAT TO SAY AND JUNK.....AND, YOU KNOW, LIKE IT'S REALLY WEIRD BUT TWELVE YEARS OF PUBLIC EDUCATION — I MEAN, WHOA!.....ANYWAY, THAT'S WHAT I THINK IN MY HEAD, YOU KNOW?"

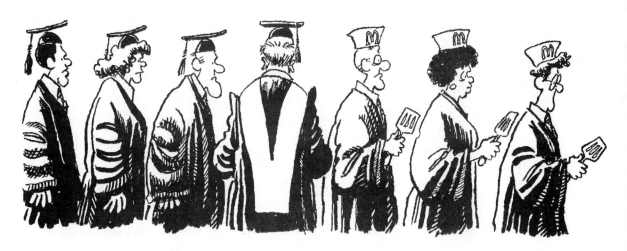

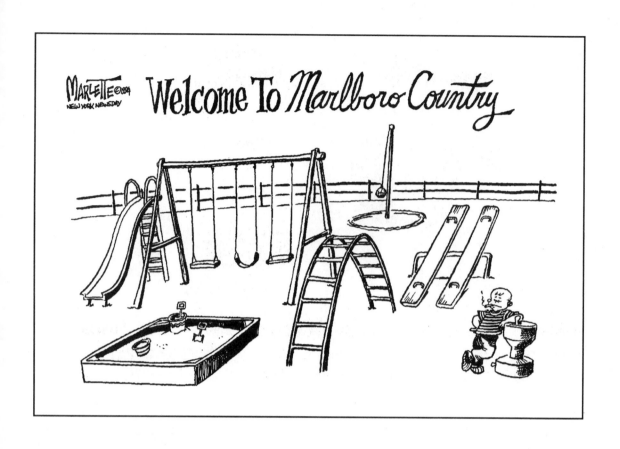

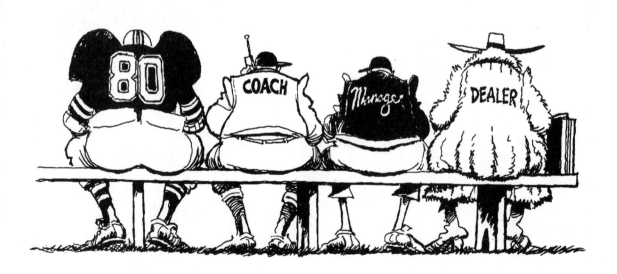

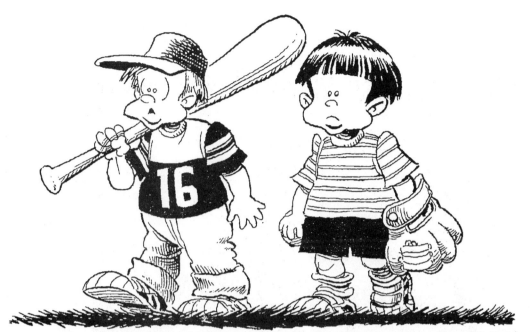

"MY PARENTS SAY IF THEY EVER CATCH ME DOING DRUGS THEY'LL KILL ME—
BUT I DON'T KNOW IF THAT'S THEM OR THE ALCOHOL TALKING!"

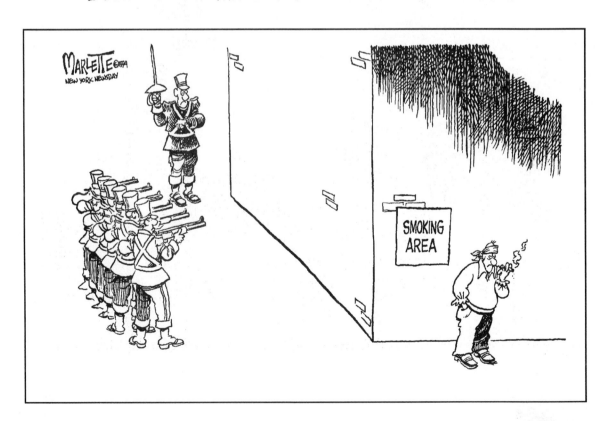

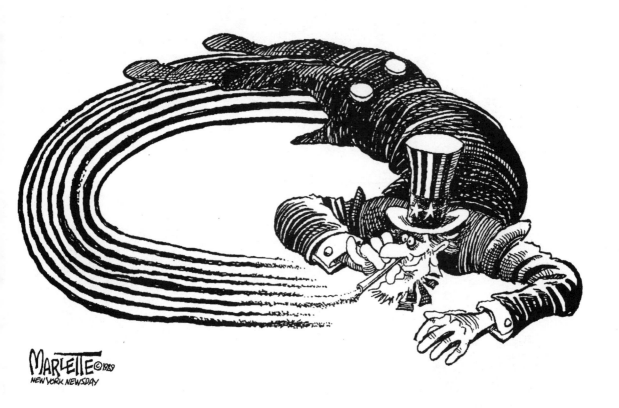

MARLETTE © 1989
NEW YORK NEWSDAY

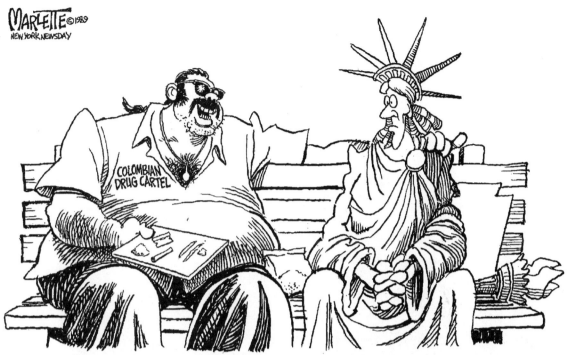

"YOUR LIPS SAY 'NO, NO', BUT YOUR NOSE SAYS 'YES, YES'!"

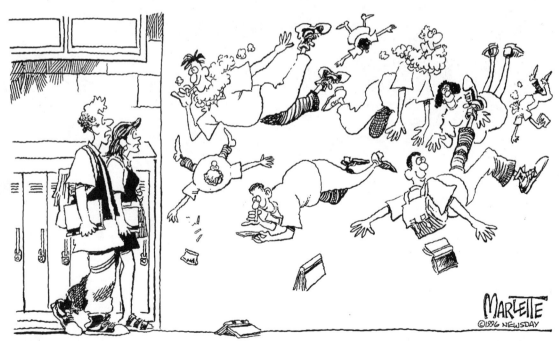

"SO THIS IS WHY THEY CALL IT *HIGH SCHOOL!*"

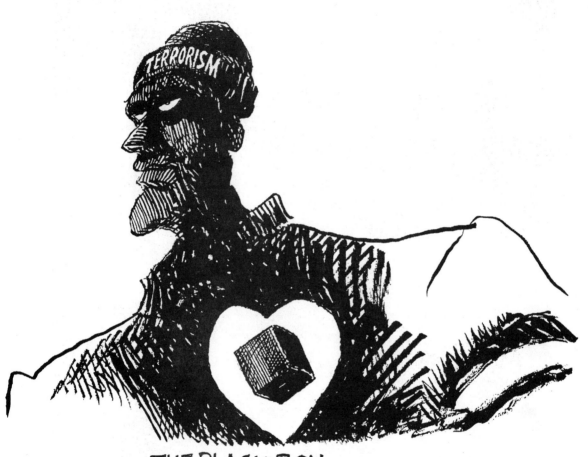

THE BLACK BOX

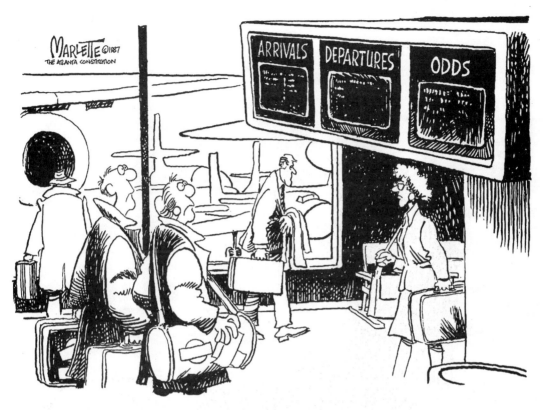

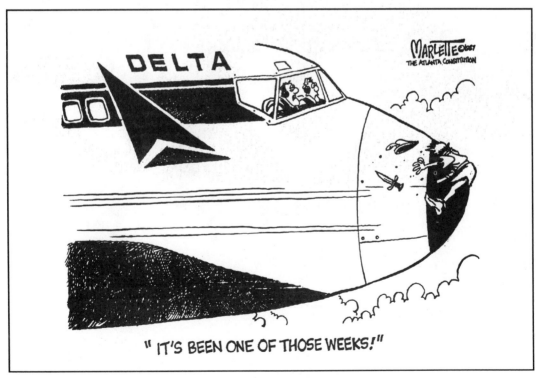

" IT'S BEEN ONE OF THOSE WEEKS!"

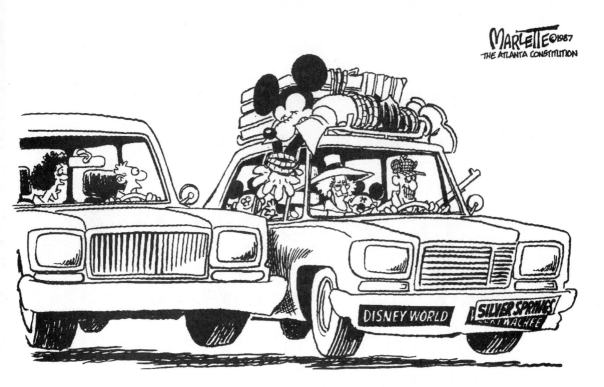

"I TOLD YOU FLORIDA NEVER SHOULD HAVE RELAXED ITS GUN LAWS!..."

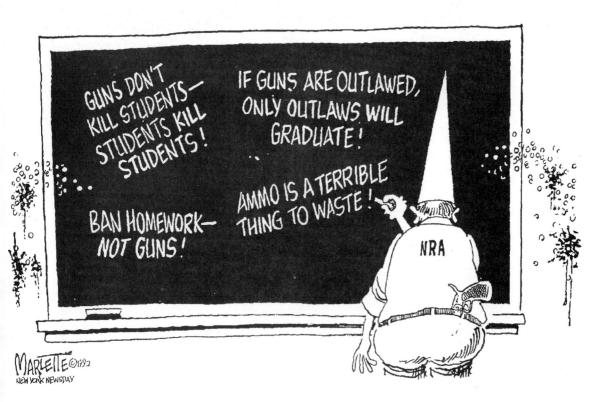

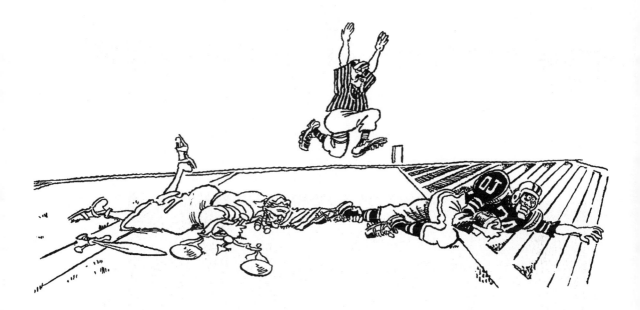

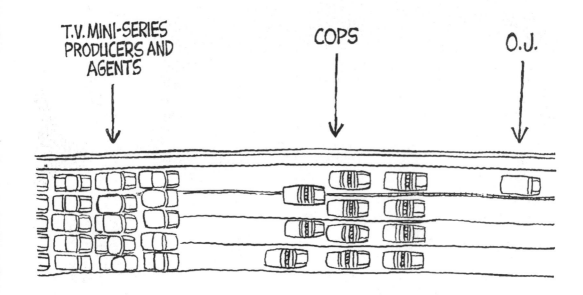

T.V. MINI-SERIES PRODUCERS AND AGENTS

COPS

O.J.

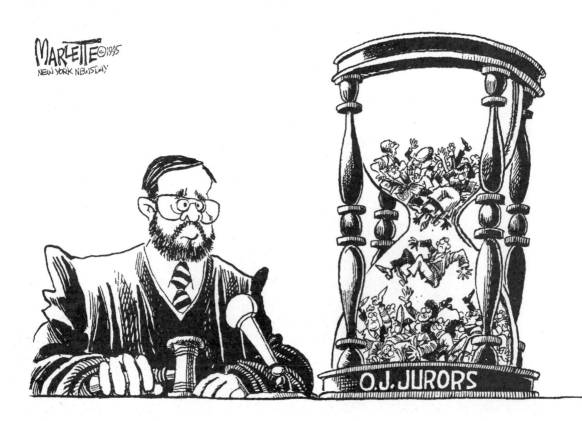

MARLETTE ©1995
NEW YORK NEWSDAY

O.J. JURORS

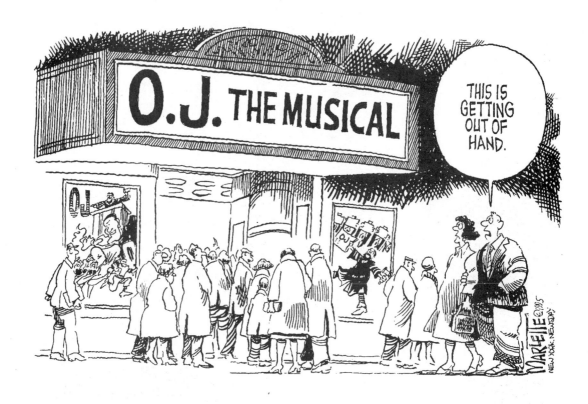

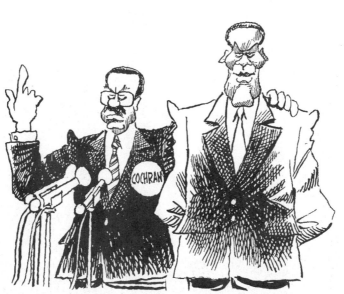

"I HAVE A DREAM THAT MY CLIENTS WILL ONE DAY LIVE IN A NATION WHERE THEY WILL NOT BE JUDGED BY THE CONTENT OF THEIR CHARACTER BUT BY THE COLOR OF THEIR SKIN!"

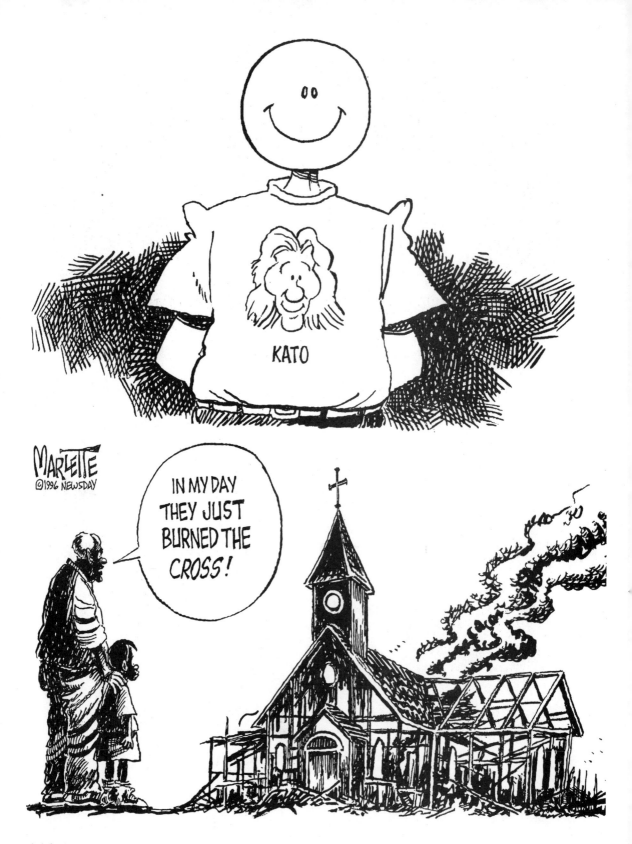

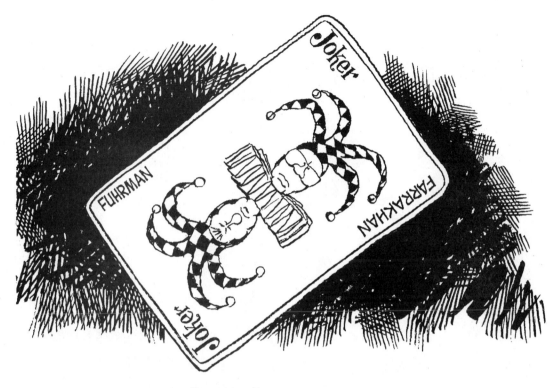

RACE CARD

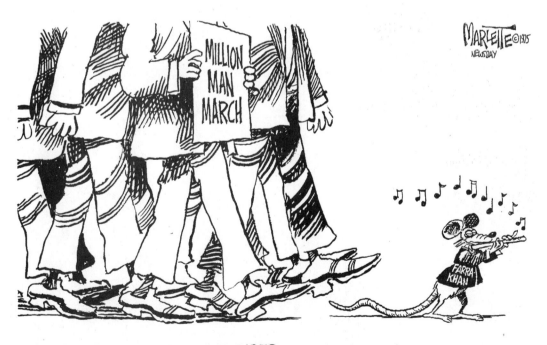

PIED PIPER

147

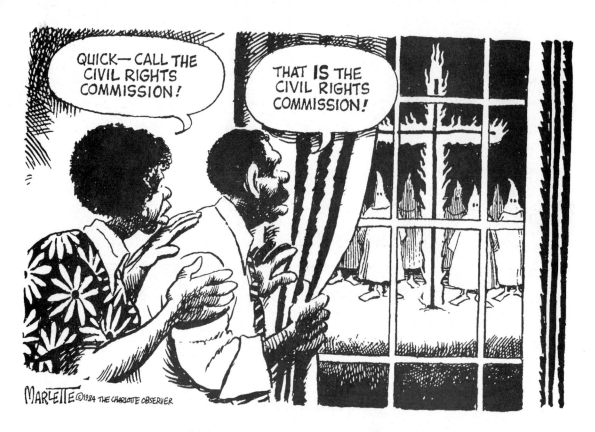

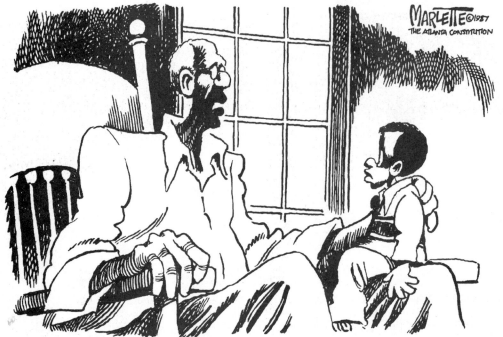

"PRESIDENT?... NO, CHILD, BUT YOU CAN GROW UP TO BE FRONT-RUNNER!"

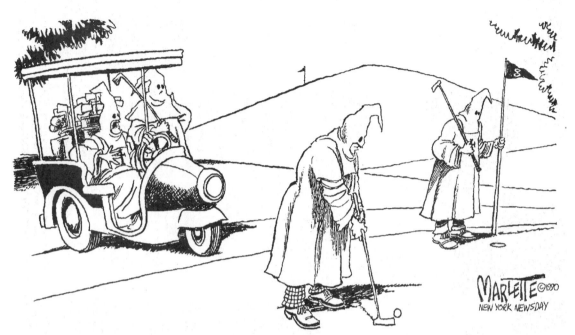

"...I MEAN, LET'S FACE IT—THE REASON YOU JOIN A COUNTRY CLUB IN THE FIRST PLACE IS SO YOU CAN MIX WITH YOUR OWN KIND!"

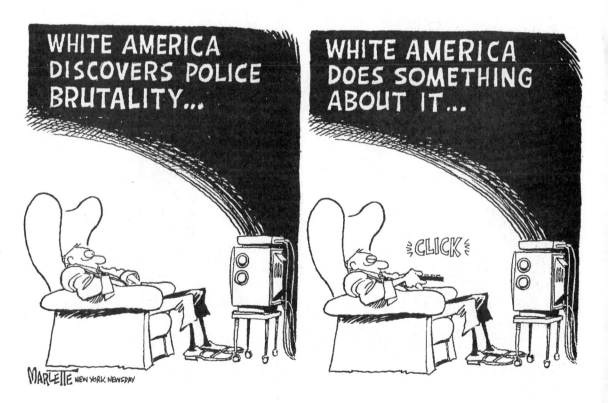

WHITE AMERICA DISCOVERS POLICE BRUTALITY...

WHITE AMERICA DOES SOMETHING ABOUT IT...

CLICK

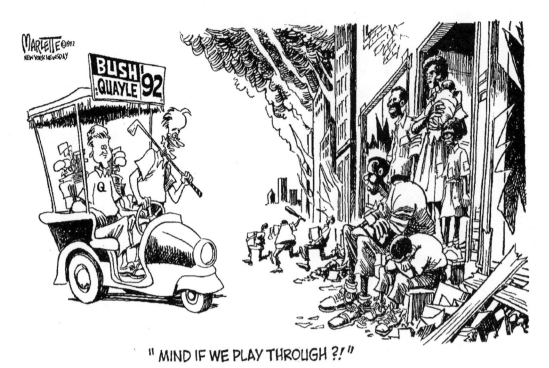

" MIND IF WE PLAY THROUGH ?!"

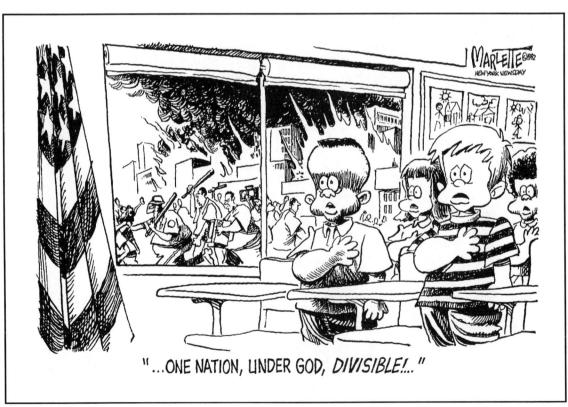

"...ONE NATION, UNDER GOD, *DIVISIBLE!...*"

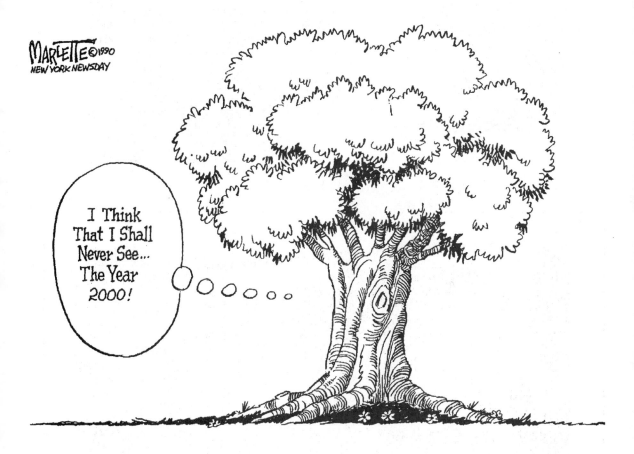

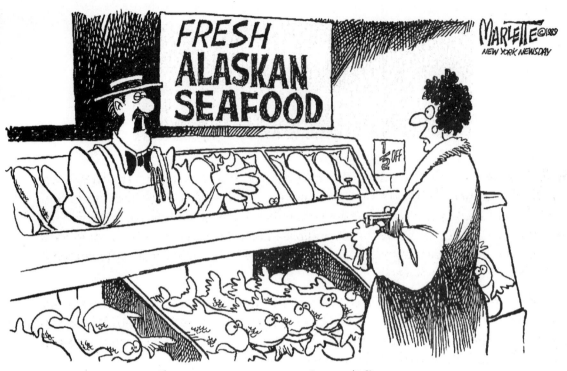

" REGULAR OR UNLEADED ? "

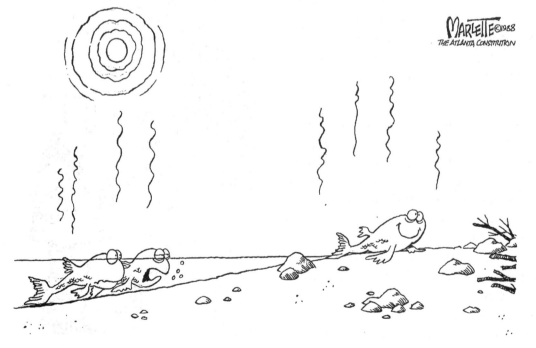

" DON'T TELL HIM IT'S THE DROUGHT— HE THINKS HE'S *EVOLVING!* "

New York: Moving to Toontown

When I told friends and family that I was moving north, they were stunned. When I said I was moving to New York City, they were horrified. I might as well have announced I was going to have a sex-change operation. They were too polite to gasp audibly and reel back in horror, but I could see it in their eyes, "You'll be mugged!" "You'll be homeless!" "You'll live in a cardboard box" "You'll become a crack dealer!"

Southerners, as a rule, are not encumbered by an exalted view of life in the big city. In fact, we are the best haters of New York City in the world—with the possible exception of New Yorkers. I have never met a Southerner who didn't have some hideous I-Loathe-New-York story to tell. Our worst paranoid nightmares about life in the city always seem to come true upon our very first visit. When Southerners come to town, we get mugged at LaGuardia's baggage claim, the cab we hail is driven by Son-of-Sam. By the time we check into our hotel, we're being sued by the Rev. Al Sharpton.

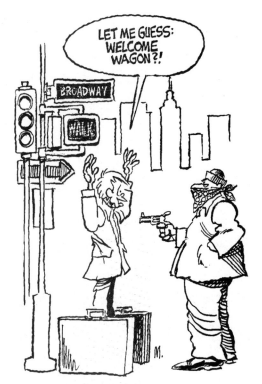

One North Carolina friend planned his first New York trip for months, arriving just in time to watch a wrecking ball and crane knock down the hotel he had been booked into. A friend from Georgia, walking down Broadway on his first visit heard a woman screaming from an apartment above the street , "Help me, Help me, He's killing me! He's killing me!" Seeing nobody heeding her calls, as any chivalrous son of the South would, he gallantly rushed into the dark building, ran up the stairs toward the screams, burst through the apartment door and into a primal-scream group therapy session. The therapist threatened to call the cops.

Within a few hours of arriving on Manhattan Island for the first time to sign my first syndication contract, I found myself being propositioned by, yes, a bisexual porno filmmaker.

Welcome to the Big Apple.

The antagonism toward New York nurtured by many southerners is primal and profound. My neighbor in Decatur, Georgia, Bruce Wilson, an attorney who has a fondness for guns, perhaps expressed it best: "I've done a lot of things in my life—some good, some not," he explained, politely declining an invitation to visit us in our new hometown. "But when I die, I hope I can look back on my life and be proud to say I never set foot in New York City."

My southern roots run deep, too, and except for a year in Cambridge, Massachusetts, on a Nieman Fellowship at Harvard, I never figured on spending much time north of the Mason-Dixon, certainly not in New York. Still, I have never mustered quite the same revulsion for Yankees or the Big Apple as some of my kinsmen.

New York's energy, excitement and vitality have always attracted me. For any artist, naturally, there is a strong gravitational pull toward New York City. It's The Show—the cultural vortex of the race, the storm center of human achievement. And it holds a special place in the dreamscapes of my youth and the mythic underpinnings of my budding ambition.

As a child growing up in small towns in North Carolina and Mississippi, I visited New York and studied its environs only from TV, movies, books and magazines. The media initiated me into the secrets, mysteries, and allures of the city.

I learned about Macy's from "Miracle on 34th Street." I knew that Rob and Laura Petrie on the "Dick Van Dyke" show lived in suburban New Rochelle. The offices of Mad magazine were located on Lexington Avenue. They made fun of admen on Madison Avenue.

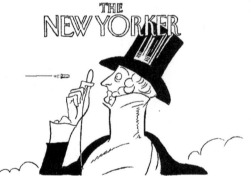

Holden Caufield and the Glass children in J.D. Salinger's novels actually traversed and grew up on the streets of Manhattan.

I saw the city through the comic prisms of Neil Simon and Woody Allen. I listened to Johnny Carson rib the Long Island Rail Road and Con Ed. Those impossibly sophisticated New Yorker cartoons informed my sense of humor.

The hip alienation and urban angst of Jule Feiffer's drawings somehow enchanted and spoke to this drawling, towheaded adolescent lost in the sweltering southern summers of my youth.

To a teenager in Mississippi, those comedians on Ed Sullivan and The Tonight Show all seemed to be sharing some wonderful inside joke with their Jewish cultural references and Yiddish expressions that I knew I would understand if only I could go to New York.

Those places and frames of reference were as much a part of the geographies of my imagination as were Judea and Samaria from my Sunday school lessons or Vicksburg and Chancellorsville from my history books. And I imbued those alien landscapes and cultures with a vitality and reality that seemed achingly absent from my own.

I sometimes compare notes and swap cracker credentials with my friend and fellow southerner, novelist Pat Conroy. He and I like to trade stories from our whiteboy roots in that trailer park of the spirit we recall as our childhood. In the wonderful tradition we artists and writers have of transforming self-pity into amusing anecdotes, we exchange stories of our up-from-slavery upbringings with a sense of stunned disbelief. We're like survivors of a genealogical plane crash, frantically going over the details in our memory, checking to make sure it really happened and we survived.

Past our prime for one-on-one basketball, we compete to see who can outdo the other with lurid recitals of family degradation and humiliation. Conroy weighs in with one of his patented yarns from his tortured youth. These usually have something to do with southern families who eat their young, as chronicled in his best-selling novels and soon to be a major motion picture.

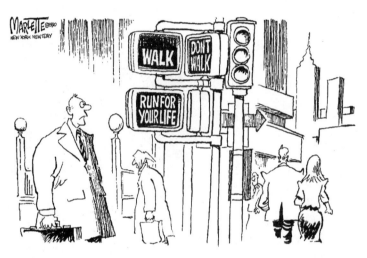

I counter with stories of my grandmother. During the Depression, my grandmother was bayoneted by a National Guardsman during a mill strike. "Mama Gracie," as we called her, dipped snuff, toted a .38 in her purse, tyrannized her family with tears and rages and would never allow us grandyoung'uns to step inside her house without taking off our shoes.

She was a virtuoso of manipulation, a museum of hysterical symptoms. She suffered psychosomatic illnesses, dreams, visions, and premonitions. A tour guide of the emotions, she specialized in the guilt trip and made sure we were all frequent

155

flyers. Like Tammy Faye Bakker, she could weep at will, and could wield that mighty weapon like a truncheon. We grandyoung'uns often prayed for a bayonet.

Mama Gracie lived in the big house and my granddaddy, her husband, lived in the little house fifteen feet from the back door of the big house. When I was a child, we'd visit her and then go out back and visit him. Granddaddy and Mama Gracie never spoke to each other, never acknowledged one another and never divorced. We grandyoung'uns joked grimly that they were staying together until the children were dead.

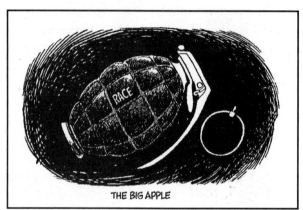

THE BIG APPLE

These two had produced eleven children together, some of whom died in infancy. Others were claimed by alcohol, drugs, madness and suicide. When one of their offspring, my uncle, actually broke out of the desperate cycle of the mill town and went off to college, even earning a master's degree, he immediately contracted a rare, incurable disease and died. Success in this family was a crime punishable by death.

Of course, in the South, colorful families are as common as barbecue joints, and a low-grade schizophrenia is the spiritual coin of the realm. Where I come from, as Faulkner reminds us, the past is not over and done. It's not even past.

Perhaps it was the vividness of the contradictions, ironies and hypocrisies in the family and culture in which I grew up that brought forth the satirist's rage and my impulse to "picture" those inconsistencies.

For whatever reasons, my professional identity has been bound up to some degree in my southerness. I won a Pulitzer Prize in part for cartoons lampooning PTL in the buckle of the Bible Belt, Charlotte, N.C. No doubt I was able to draw a bead on Jim and Tammy before it was cool because I attended Sunday school at Magnolia Street Baptist Church. I draw a comic strip, *Kudzu*, named for a vine that covers the South and set in a small southern town, Bypass—because that is what I know.

But I don't think of myself as a "southern" cartoonist, whatever that means. I have never sat down at the drawing board to chronicle the folkways and mores of Dixie—to catalog humorous and colorful items of interest from below the Mason-Dixon, like some Stuckey's souvenir shop of the funny pages. Yes, I am attracted to issues of race, religion and family. How can you grow up in the South and not be? But aren't those issues as important to midtown Manhattan and Long Island as they are to Peachpit, Georgia. Certainly they were central in the last presidential campaign.

I don't know how my move north will affect my work and the way I see things, but I'm sure they will be affected. Artists are emotional teabags. We have a semi-permeable membrane for skin. Everything gets under our skin and eventually finds its way into our work.

How does it feel to leave the South? I have long suspected Malcolm X was right:

The South is south of the Canadian border. The problems of my native region—the racism depicted by the jarring "white" and "colored" signs on the water fountains of my youth, the poverty and ignorance that crippled the spirit of the region—were just vivid symptoms of a disease that afflicts the nation as a whole. It's not very far, it turns out, from Forsyth County, Georgia, to Howard Beach.

So, in a way, I feel at home moving north. Growing up in the South in the '60s, we were the nation's scapegoat and whipping boy—we wore our private demons and public neuroses on our sleeves—and

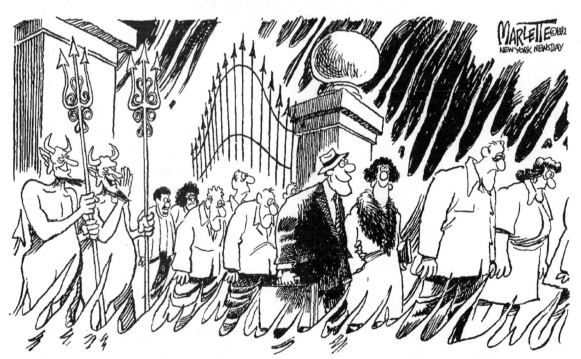

"YOU CAN ALWAYS TELL THE NEW YORKERS—THEY THINK THIS IS *HEAVEN!*"

the world had something to point at. However, I notice over the last few years that the South, as it homogenizes itself into the Sunbelt, has slowly relinquished its title, giving up its role as America's designated punching bag.

New York City, Bonfire of the Vanities, has claimed that position in the demonology of America's collective unconscious. New York-bashing is a national sport now. New York is the new Mississippi—New York Burning. For all its glitz, glamor and opportunity, the problems of modern life in the city have grown to such a scale and magnitude—drugs, homelessness, greed, corruption—that New York has become what Mississippi was in the '60s—America's problem child, the scapegoat, a mess.

The issues loom large in this urban crucible. The problems are clear and easy to see. Like the setting of my southern childhood, the contradictions and ironies and hypocrisies are vivid. They stand out in stark and stunning relief. It's all a caricature—a cartoon, really. New York City is Toontown. This southerner should feel right at home.

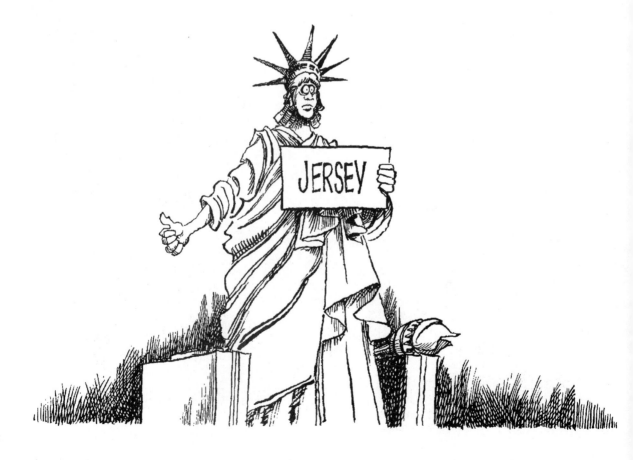

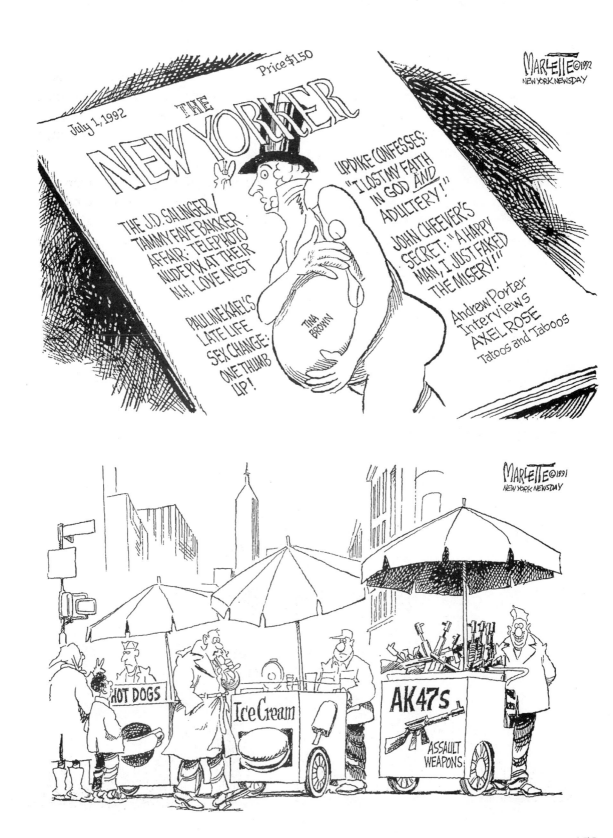

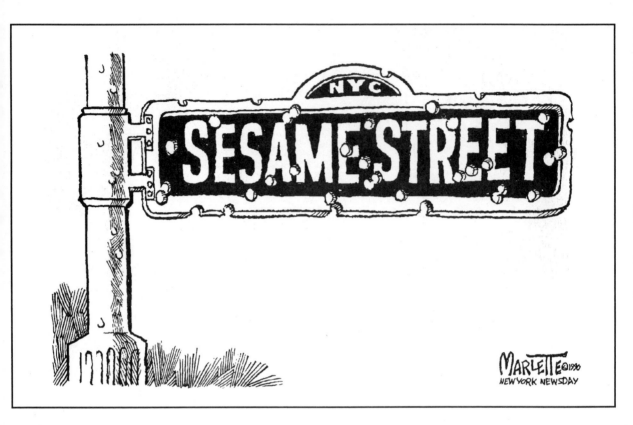

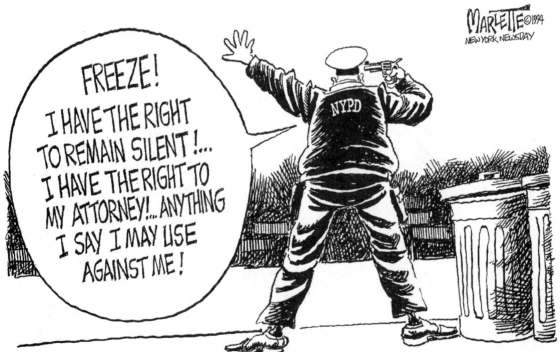

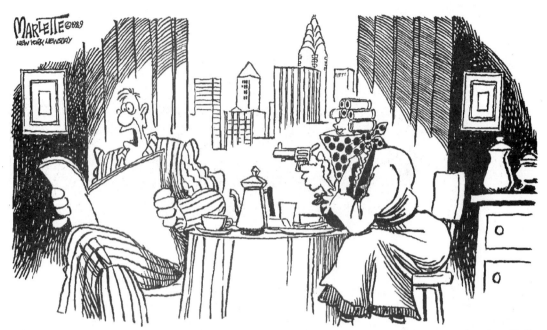

"LISTEN TO THIS POLL, HONEY— LAST YEAR ONE OUT OF TWO NEW YORKERS WERE VICTIMS OF CRIME!"

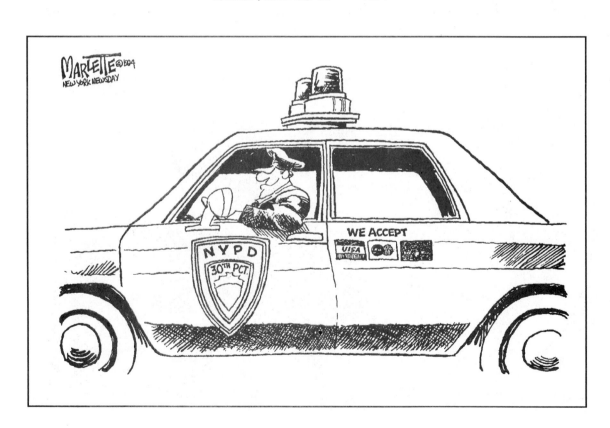

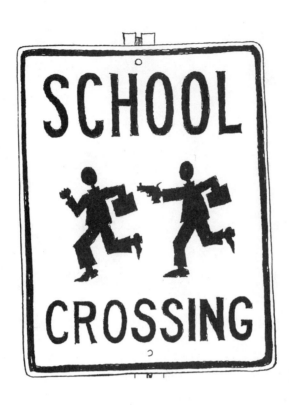

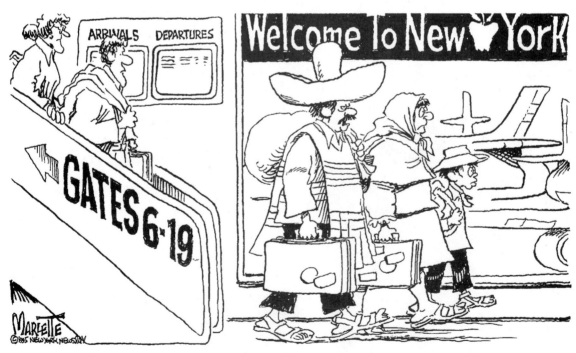

"WHATEVER YOU DO, DON'T DRINK THE WATER!"

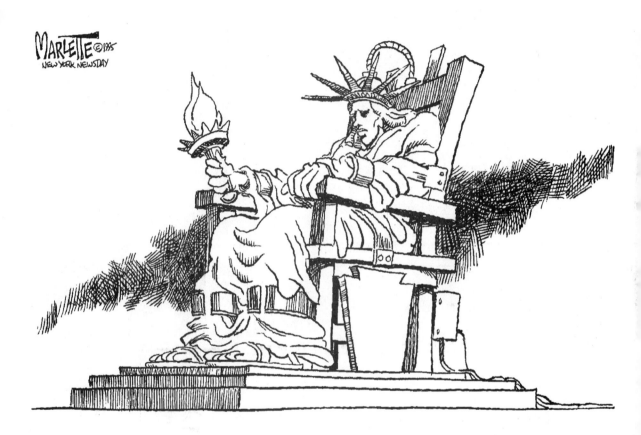

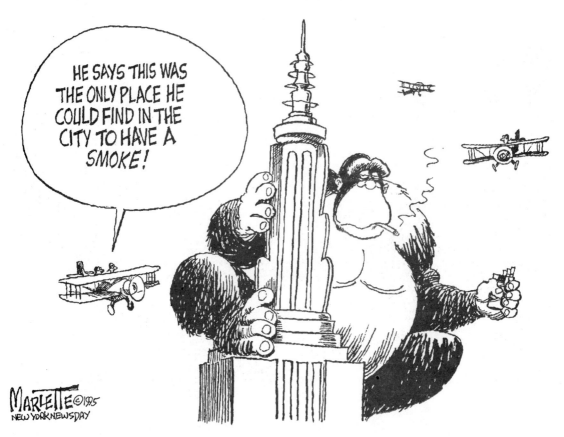

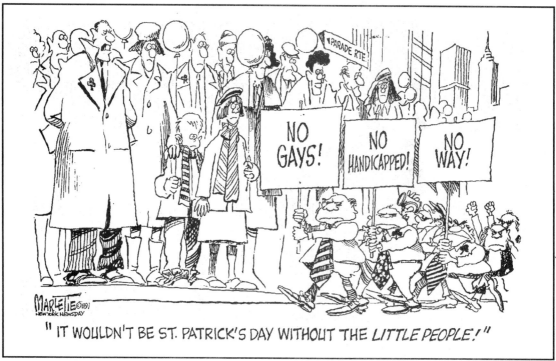

"IT WOULDN'T BE ST. PATRICK'S DAY WITHOUT THE *LITTLE PEOPLE!*"

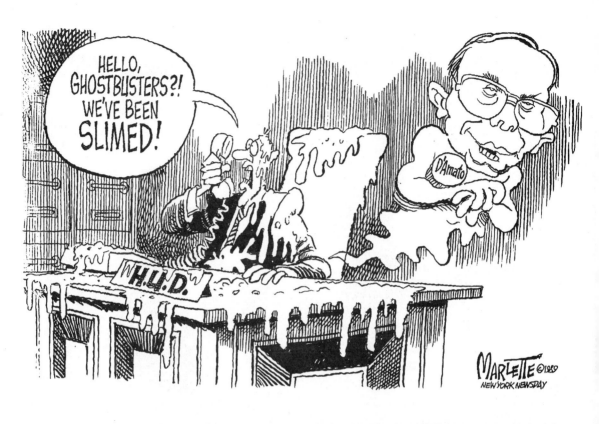

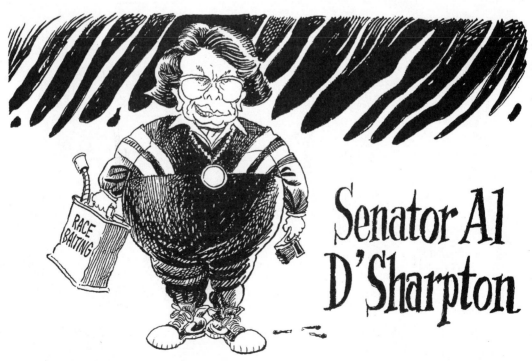

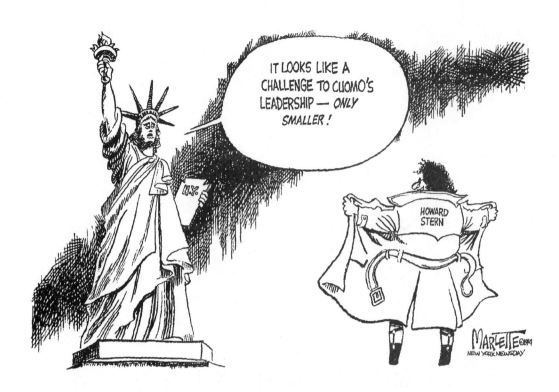

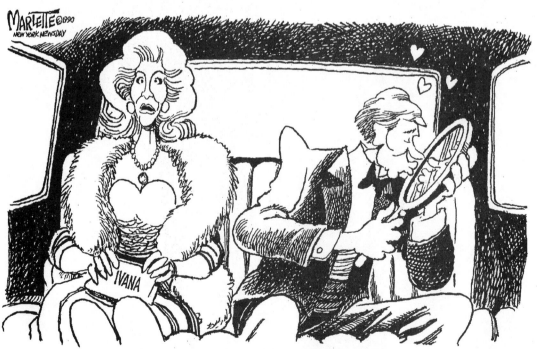

"THERE'S SOMEONE ELSE, ISN'T THERE, DONALD?!"

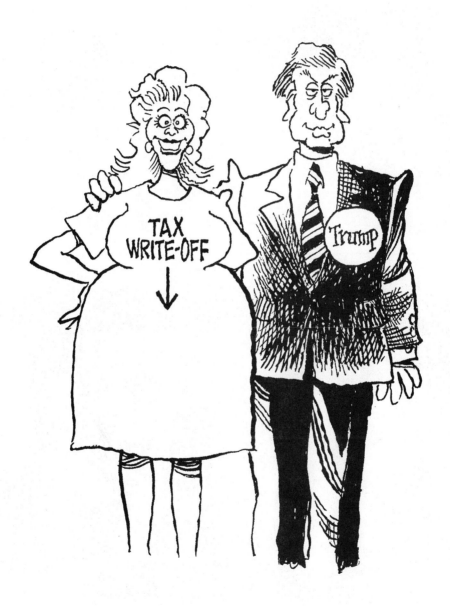

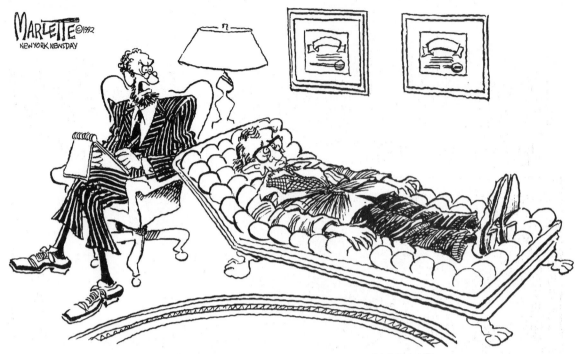

"WHY, THAT'S THE *SICKEST* THING I EVER HEARD!"

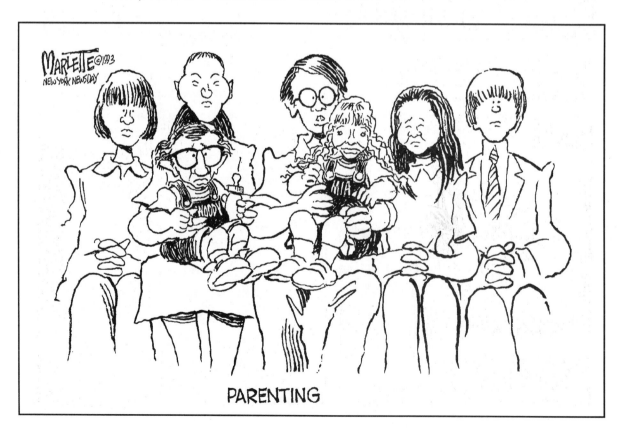

PARENTING

My FIRST New York Dinner Party!
by DOUG MARLETTE — TRANSPLANTED SOUTHERNER

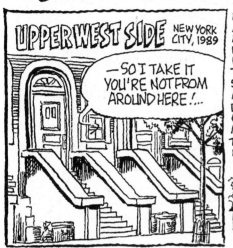

UPPER WEST SIDE — NEW YORK CITY, 1989

—SO I TAKE IT YOU'RE NOT FROM AROUND HERE.!...

MY INTERROGATOR, A SOPHISTICATED, MIDDLE-AGED LADY WITH A VAGUELY BRITISH LILT TO HER TONGUE, WAS SEATED NEXT TO ME AT AN ELEGANT DINNER GATHERING GIVEN TO WELCOME ME AND MY FAMILY TO OUR BROWNSTONE NEIGHBORHOOD...

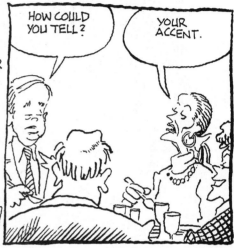

HOW COULD YOU TELL?

YOUR ACCENT.

IN MANHATTAN YOU QUICKLY LEARN THAT WHEN YOU OPEN YOUR MOUTH AND SPEAK WITH A SOUTHERN DRAWL YOUR I.Q. AUTOMATICALLY DROPS BELOW ROOM TEMPERATURE...

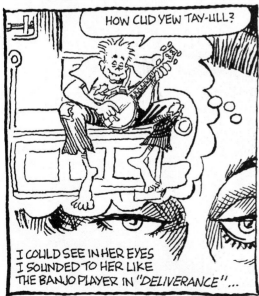

HOW CUD YEW TAY-ULL?

I COULD SEE IN HER EYES I SOUNDED TO HER LIKE THE BANJO PLAYER IN "DELIVERANCE"...

SHE MOVED IN FOR THE KILL:

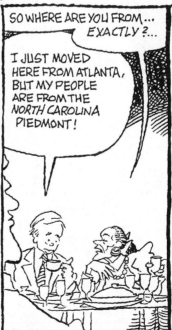

SO WHERE ARE YOU FROM... EXACTLY?...

I JUST MOVED HERE FROM ATLANTA, BUT MY PEOPLE ARE FROM THE NORTH CAROLINA PIEDMONT!

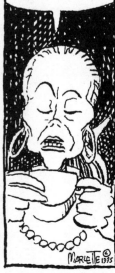

OOOH! I DON'T SEE HOW ANYBODY COULD POSSIBLY LIVE DOWN THERE WITH THOSE PEOPLE!

MARLETTE © 1995

169

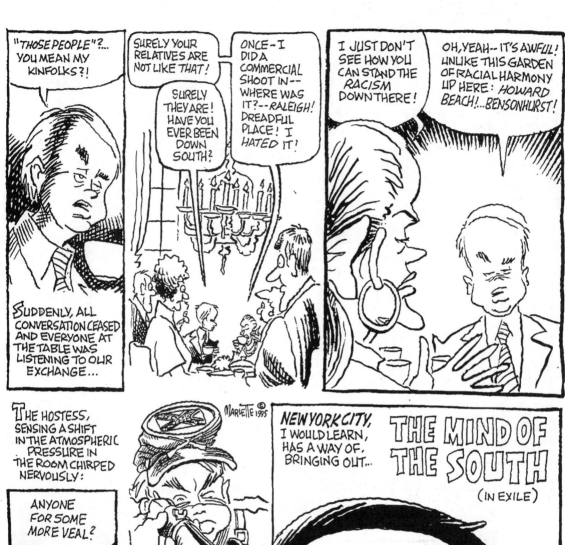

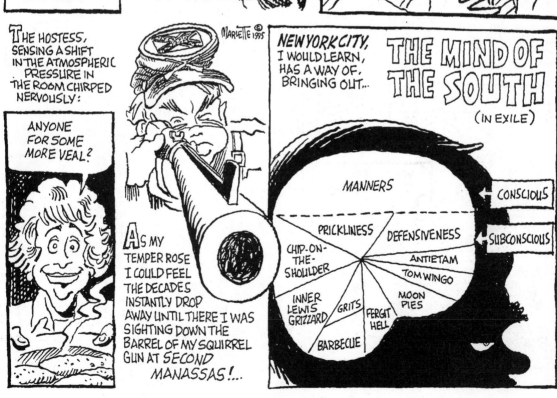

MEANWHILE, BACK AT THE SOIREE:

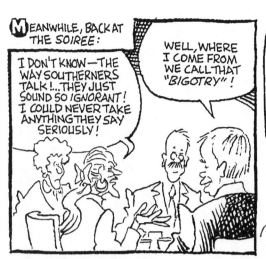

I DON'T KNOW—THE WAY SOUTHERNERS TALK!...THEY JUST SOUND SO *IGNORANT*! I COULD NEVER TAKE ANYTHING THEY SAY *SERIOUSLY*!

WELL, WHERE I COME FROM WE CALL THAT "*BIGOTRY*"!

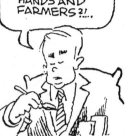

TRUE, MY PEOPLE WERE RACISTS, BUT WHAT DO YOU EXPECT FROM UNEDUCATED, POOR, SMALL-TOWN MILL-HANDS AND FARMERS?!...

"...AT LEAST THEY HAD AN EXCUSE FOR THEIR NARROW-MINDED PROVINCIALISM!... THEY WERE *DEPRIVED*!

GEN. SHERMAN THE PLAZA

"I MEET NEW YORKERS WHO HAVE EVERY ADVANTAGE, CULTURAL AND EDUCATIONAL, BUT FOR ALL THEIR PRIVILEGE AND ERUDITION THEY'RE THE MOST PREJUDICED, CLOSE-MINDED AND PROVINCIAL SUCKERS I EVER SAW!"

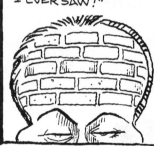

" RULE *NUMBER ONE* HERE IN *NEW YORK*: '*DON'T LOOK!*'

YO! CHECK IT OUT!

PSSST! BUDDY!

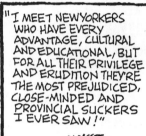

...YOU WALK FAST DOWN THE STREET, EYES STRAIGHT AHEAD..."

"IT'S SELF-PRESERVATION, SURE, BUT Y'ALL SEEM TO GO THROUGH LIFE THAT WAY—WITH *BLINDERS*!"

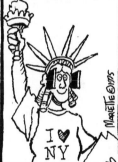

I ♥ NY

IN THE SOUTH IGNORANCE IS AN AFFLICTION— IN *NEW YORK* IT'S A CHOICE!

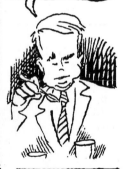

BY NOW, THE HOSTESS WAS BESIDE HERSELF:

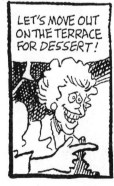

LET'S MOVE OUT ON THE TERRACE FOR DESSERT!

WELL, I HOPE I DIDN'T OFFEND.

JUST CURIOUS— YOUR ACCENT... WHERE ARE YOU FROM?

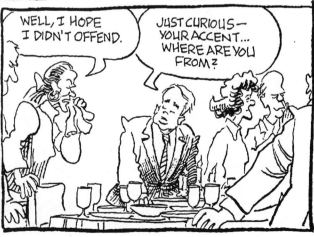

SOUTH AFRICA

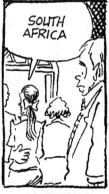

AS WE SAY IN NEW YORK, "*TRUE STORY!*"

171

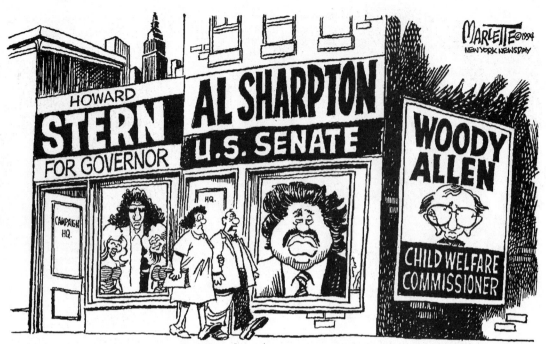

"THAT'S IT—ONE MORE THING AND I'M MOVING TO JERSEY!"

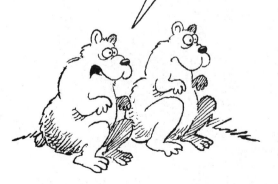

LEGEND HAS IT THAT IF HE COMES OUT AND SEES HIS SHADOW WE'LL GET FOUR MORE YEARS OF *MARIO!*

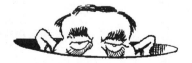

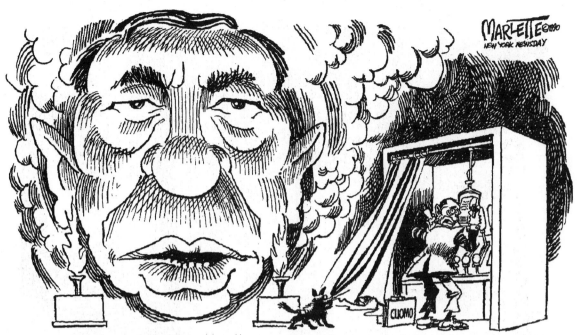

"THE GREAT AND GLORIOUS OZ HAS SPOKEN!... PAY NO ATTENTION TO THE MAN BEHIND THE CURTAIN!..."

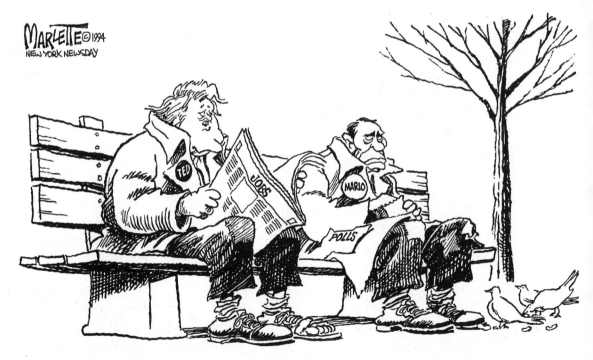

"JUST THINK—TEN YEARS AGO THIS WOULD HAVE BEEN A *DREAM TICKET!...*"

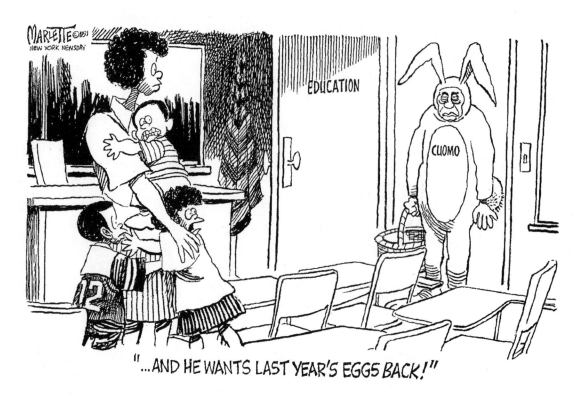

"...AND HE WANTS LAST YEAR'S EGGS BACK!"

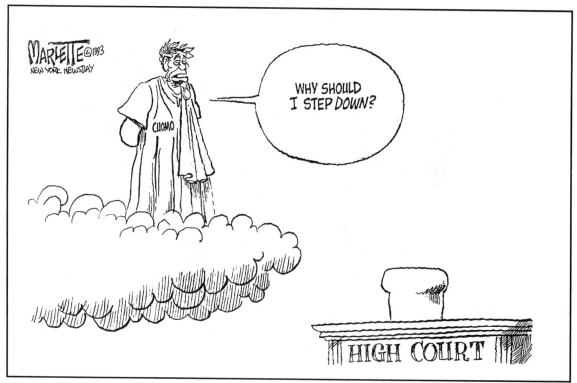

WHY SHOULD I STEP *DOWN*?

HIGH COURT

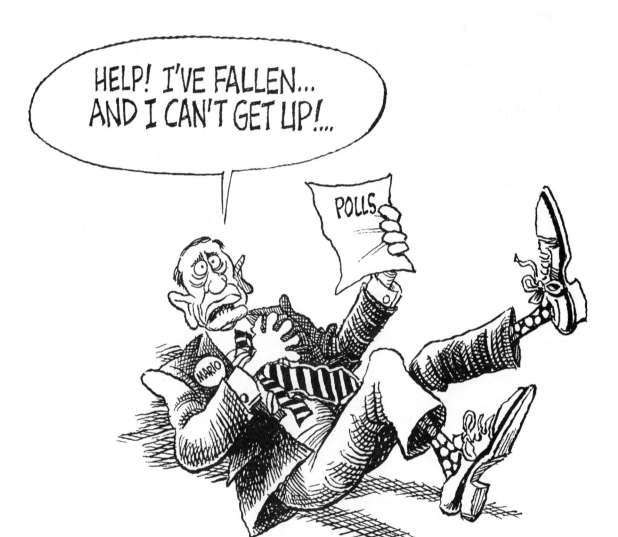

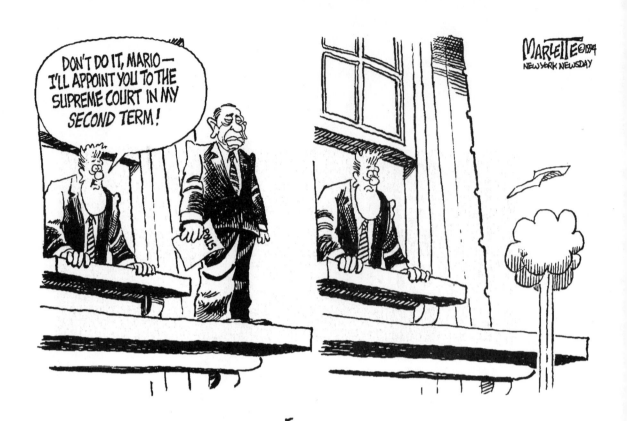

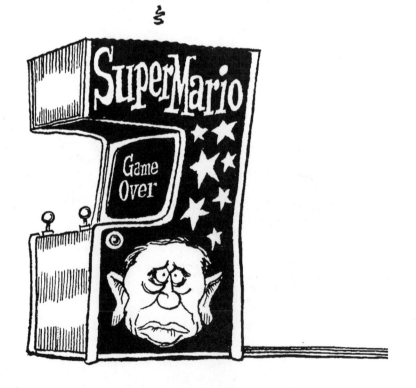

Happy Trails:
Obituary Cartoons

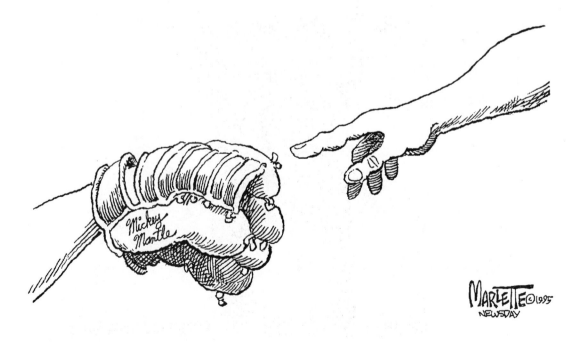

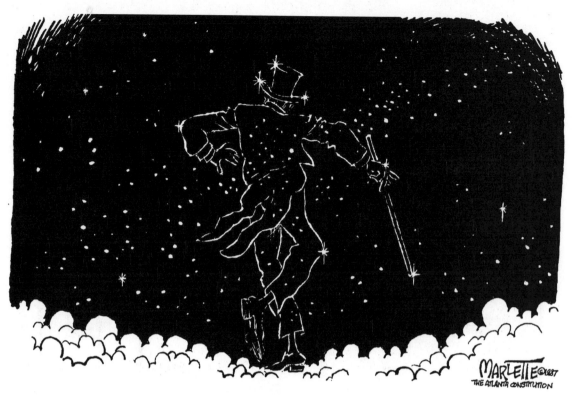

TOP HAT

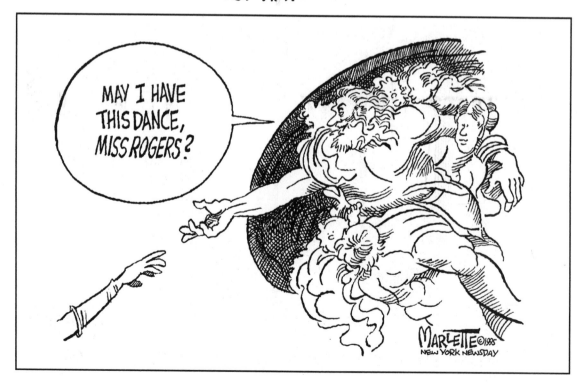

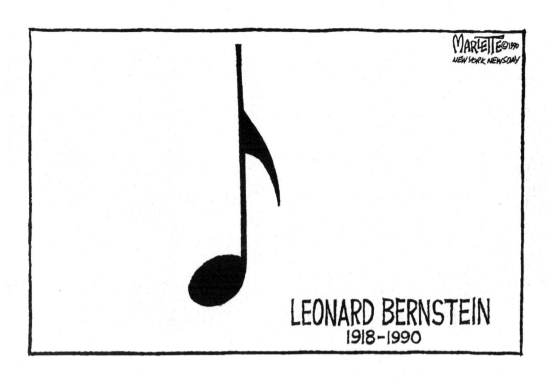

LEONARD BERNSTEIN
1918-1990

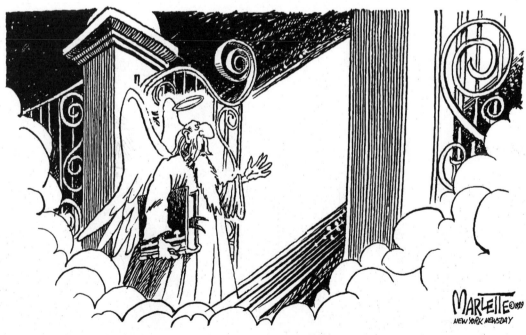

" RELAX—EVERYBODY'S NERVOUS PLAYING OPPOSITE *OLIVIER!* "

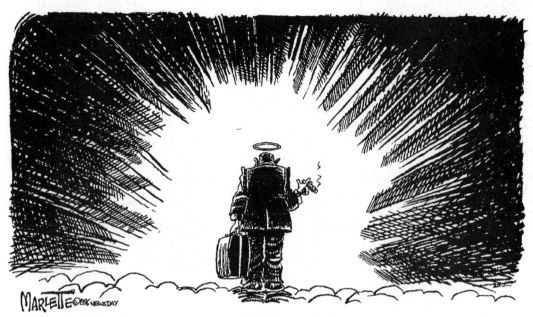

"GRACIE, I GOT THE PART!"

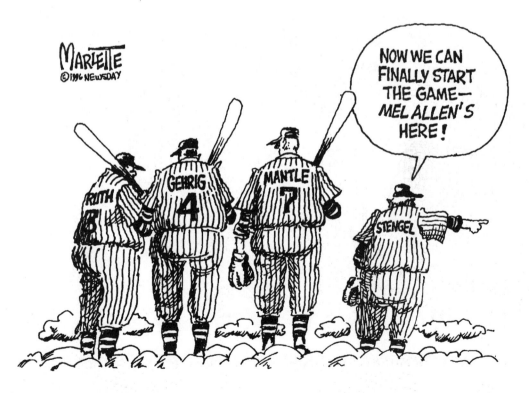

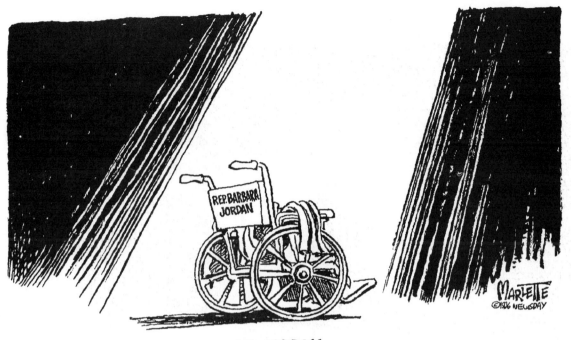

AIR JORDAN

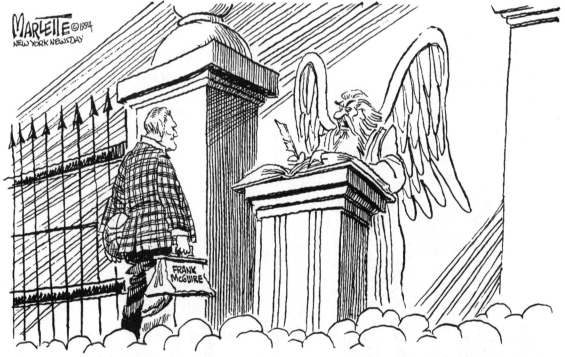

"WHAT DO YOU MEAN FROM NOW ON YOU'LL HANDLE ALL THE RECRUITING FROM NEW YORK CITY?!"

Jacqueline Kennedy Onassis

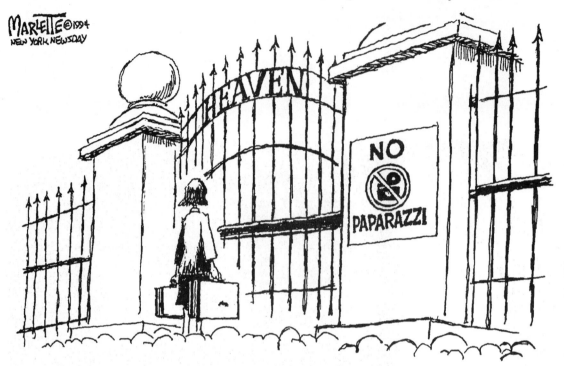

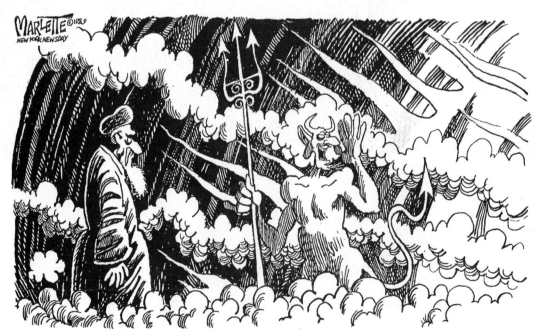

" MAKE ROOM FOR ANOTHER *HOLY MAN!* "

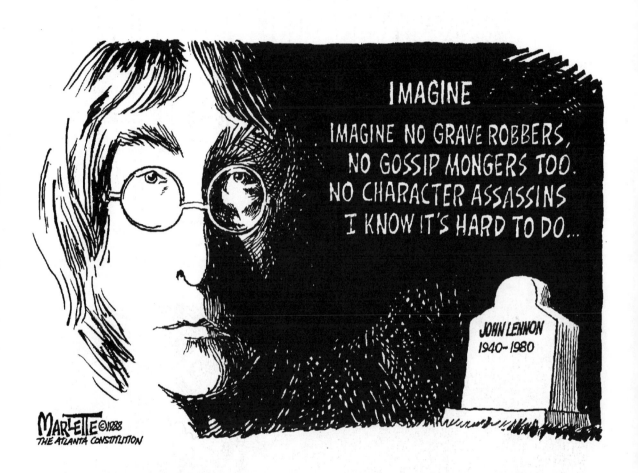

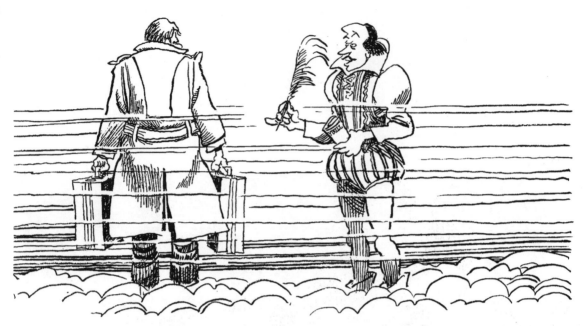

"WOULD YOU SIGN MY PLAYBILL, MR. PAPP?"

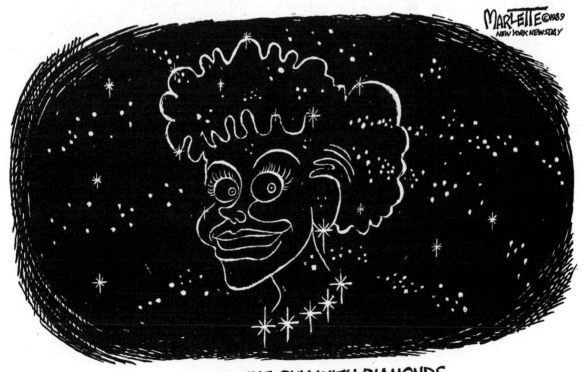

LUCY IN THE SKY WITH DIAMONDS

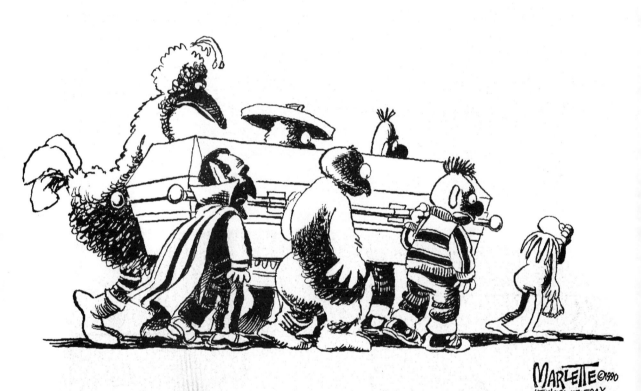